~~NOT~~ ~~A DIET~~ ~~BOOK~~

JAMES SMITH

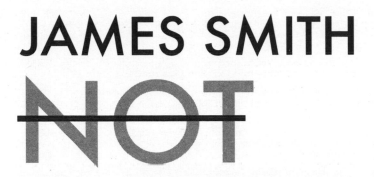
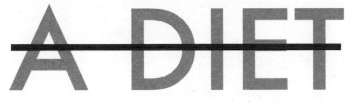
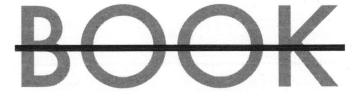

NOT A DIET BOOK

TAKE CONTROL.
GAIN CONFIDENCE.
CHANGE YOUR LIFE.

HarperCollins*Publishers*

p.20 Extract from *The 4-Hour Work Week* by Tim Ferriss. Reproduced by permission of The Random House Group Limited. Copyright © Tim Ferriss, 2011. And by permission of Crown Books, an imprint of Random House, a division of Penguin Random House LLC. Copyright © Tim Ferriss 2007, 2009 by Carmenere One, LLC.

p. 73 Extract from *The Story of Philosophy* by Will Durant. Reproduced by permission of SSA, a division of Simon & Schuster, Inc. Copyright © Will Durant, 1961.

p.77 Extract from *Atomic Habits* by James Clear. Reproduced by permission of The Random House Group Limited and by permission of Avery, an imprint of Penguin Publishing Group, a division of Penguin Random House, LLC. Copyright © James Clear, 2018.

p.99 and 107 Extracts from *Why We Sleep* by Matthew Walker. Reproduced by permission of Penguin Books Ltd. and by of permission of Scribner, a division of Simon & Schuster, Inc. Copyright © Matthew Walker, 2017.

p. 129 and 144 Extracts from *The Subtle Art of Not Giving a F*ck* by Mark Manson. Reproduced by permission of HarperCollins Publishers and Pan Macmillian Australia Pty Ltd. Copyright © Mark Manson, 2016.

p.158 and 161 Extracts from *Ego is the Enemy* by Ryan Holiday. Reproduced by permission of Profile Books. Copyright © Ryan Holiday, 2017.

HarperCollins*Publishers*
1 London Bridge Street
London SE1 9GF

www.harpercollins.co.uk

First published by HarperCollins*Publishers* 2020
This paperback edition published 2020

10 9 8 7 6 5 4 3 2 1

© James Smith 2020

James Smith asserts the moral right to be identified as the author of this work

A catalogue record of this book is available from the British Library

ISBN 978-0-00-837429-7

Printed and bound in Great Britain by CPI Group (UK) Ltd, Croydon

Contents

Foreword   vii

PART I: FOUNDATIONS

Introduction   3
A Brief History of James Smith   19

Consumer – Method – Principle   25
The Calorie Deficit   37
Fitness 'Tracking' and NEATUP247   59
Habits   73
Essentials for the Good Life   87
Understanding Diabetes Mellitus – For Everyone   111
Laws of the Universe   119
The Power of Numbers   131
Polarization   135
Effort and Ambition   139
Effort 2.0   149

PART II: BUILDING ON YOUR FOUNDATIONS

Somatotypes and Sport Selection   171
Fitness Fallacies   181
Female Fat Loss   261

Not the End   279

References   285
Acknowledgements   289
Further Reading   291
Index   293

Foreword

I know from experience that many books are never finished by the reader. They might be purchased as a gift, or at the airport before a flight; you may commit to the first chapter, but before you know it the book has become an ornament, gathering dust on your bedside table. Each day you see these books, and a little part of you tells a lie that one day you'll finish them. The collection only grows over time, and you'll usually tell yourself something along the lines of: 'I'm doing pretty well, so I don't really need to read them right now.'

I didn't read a book from start to finish until I was twenty-seven years old. I'm not someone with an academic background, and it didn't come naturally to me; but in the last few years, books have been essential in changing, sculpting and building my mindset, attitude and approach to many things – from lifestyle to relationships and my work life.

And, to be completely honest with you, writing this book was not difficult. If anything, I have so much I want to teach you that I wasn't sure I was going to fit it all in one book, so believe me when I tell you this: every single chapter in this book can affect your life in a positive way – but only if you choose to read them. Nothing is in here just to make up the word count; it's all important, and with every single page I have had you in mind – your problems, your struggles and what I can teach you to make them go away.

For each of you, somewhere in this book is one simple sentence that will revolutionize your life for ever. However, that sentence is utterly powerless until you make the decision to read it. What I have written cannot help you if this book joins all the others – the unread ornaments.

I have written this book not for me, but for you. It's all here – everything you need to begin a new chapter of your life. You'll have a new lease of clarity to take with you every day, enough understanding to make change, not just in the gym, but in your relationships, your professional life and your general perception of the people around you.

I am confident when I say that when you turn the last page of this book your life will be different. You'll be more knowledgeable, more confident and more in control.

For those of you who may not finish the book, I believe you would be doing yourself and those around you a disservice. It is here to empower you, so if there is just one book you commit to finishing, let it be this one.

Quite simply, after this, things won't be the same.

Are you ready? Let's begin.

James

PART I
FOUNDATIONS

Introduction

The first part of this book may be a little different from what you expect. At least I hope it is. Because if you've picked it up, I assume you're intending to achieve genuine, long-lasting change that will improve all areas of your life for good. So this is not the latest fitness trend or diet fad packaged up in book form to give it validity. And with this in mind, it's important to set solid foundations before thinking or talking about what the end result is going to look like. In the coming chapters I am going to wipe the slate clean for you, eliminating all the unhelpful diet myths, fads and misinformation, and reset your thinking, so you can start to identify how your future is going to look and even how it's going to feel.

With each new page, we will examine why perhaps you haven't accomplished what you've set out to do before. I very much doubt this book is the first of your efforts towards a healthier, better-balanced lifestyle. And while it may seem a bit tedious to read an entire book when there's inevitably a one-size-fits-all plan on offer on Instagram, you need to trust me here: you have to walk before you can run, and if it was that simple to make lasting change, I wouldn't have needed to write a book. But once you have come to the end of it, you should no longer need me – everything will slot into place and you'll be ready to begin living the life you've always wanted and achieving your goals.

'Give me six hours to chop down a tree and I will spend the first four hours sharpening the axe.'

Abraham Lincoln

REFERENCING

Throughout the book, I have referenced studies – if you wish to know more about these, you can search online for the full text (see p.285). Many of these link to other studies when discussing certain claims or topics; this is handy for anyone who wants to go down the rabbit hole of any relevant data that's been collated. I have also provided a Further Reading list (see p.291), which I strongly recommend getting on top of.

The fitness industry right now

There are industries all over the world designed to give consumers what they want or need for an easier or better life. For instance, the automotive industry allows us to buy various transportation methods, such as cars, for commuting or transporting the family around. It's an industry that serves a purpose, and even though consumers are aware that there is a mark-up on the goods, they don't mind because they are getting a solution to their transportation problem: for the price they pay they gain freedom, control and enjoyment, and they generally trust the provider – a win-win situation. This fairly straightforward analogy highlights the problems with the fitness industry – people are more desperate than ever for a solution to their health and fitness problems, but they are being misled and mis-sold the dream by organizations profiteering from the consumer remaining in the dark about how to help themselves, especially when it comes to fat loss.

The fitness industry should be about showing people what the human body can accomplish. It should be there to motivate the sedentary to get more from their bodies, the one shell they spend their entire lives in. Imagine if you knew you could only have one car for the rest of your life; would you take better care of it? That should be the message to send people to inspire them when they're not sure about whether to train or not. When people have a health scare or see a photo of themselves that deflates and depresses them, they should have the fitness industry to turn to for salvation.

Gyms should be full of motivated members, with experienced trainers at their disposal to provide guidance and expertise, making them feel incredibly comfortable during their first ever gym experience and beyond. There should be dietitians advising on specialist nutritional needs. And there should be a plethora of accurate scientific and evidence-based guidelines to follow, so that as new discoveries are made in the field of nutrition and training, the consumer can make small adjustments to ensure they get the most out of their time in the gym and outside of it. It'd be nice for government recommendations to be more helpful too; isn't it funny that different nations have different 'guidelines' for their populations, although they share a common obesity issue?

Diet fads should be laughed at by consumers who fully understand the mechanism behind fat loss. 'No thanks' should be the answer to anyone trying to promote celery-juice cleanses and cabbage-soup diets and those selling aloe vera (formerly aftersun) as a solution to fat loss.

Each and every one of us should know roughly how much we need to eat to remain in shape. We should have a vague idea of our daily calorie needs. We should all dip in and out of tracking our food in periods when we gain a bit of weight and enjoy *not* restricting when we're not seeking compositional change. Weight gain will not be scrutinized or demonized because we will know how to lose the weight we have gained. We should be able to pick up an item of food and consider its caloric value and the weight it has against our intake, so that we can play around social occasions, in the same way that we might with our finances. So it should work in the same way that it does when you pick up a designer watch or handbag – your brain being able to budget whether or not you can afford it based on your payslip and upcoming bills. By no means should it be like the 'matrix', where someone picks up a potato and sees binary code dictating whether or not they should consume it that day, but the frontal lobe of anyone's brain should at least be able to make a close estimate of how much they are eating each day and the decisions they need to make if they don't want to exceed their appropriate calorie intake.

This is not obsessive; it's calculative. However, if this was already the case throughout the fitness industry, I wouldn't be writing this book.

Unfortunately, the current state of the fitness industry is a far cry from my utopian description. It's in dire straits – and the worst thing is that the extent of the problem, I believe, is not fully known by the general public, many of whom are handing over large percentages of their disposable income to expensive gym memberships, diet plans, supplements, unsustainable diet fads and 'miracle' fat-loss drinks.

Doctors, lawyers and, in fact, people in most professions can face legal repercussions for what could be deemed as 'bad advice' or even 'malpractice'. However, there is very little regulation within the fitness industry, no repercussions for influencers misleading someone or giving terrible advice. This has made it a free for all for 'experts' on social media, their blue-tick gravitas making it easy to mass-market poor information, leaving the people who need help the most further disheartened, frustrated and unsure where to turn for good advice. At the time of writing, no qualifications are required to promote supplements, diets or even injectable fat-loss solutions on social media to an audience that could easily include young, impressionable teenagers, as well as older generations. This is a serious symptom of the fitness industry's – my industry's – currently broken state.

The consumer ends up trusting someone with a lot of followers and a blue tick on Instagram whom they believe to be giving expert advice, which, more often than not, is simply not the case. I know that I fit my own 'blue tick' description, but this platform is rife with people who have built a large following based on very little expertise – simply from years (or sometimes only months) of taking their tops off in photos for 'double taps' or manipulating the viral nature of current trends.

In time, the social-media 'influencer' gains gravitas, not only for sponsorship opportunities (#AD), but also with consumers – people looking for help, who make the assumption: 'Wow, they have a large following, so they must be trustworthy.'

There is also another trend to put someone on a prime-time TV show who's going to cause the biggest backlash on Twitter. And it has more to do with eliciting a response – any response – from viewers than it has to do with good information.

The industry is loaded with people with poor qualifications and little to no experience, whose only goal is to capitalize on their time in the limelight. These people are more concerned with their next payslip from their #AD campaign. The one-size-fits-all gimmick leaves the consumer deflated; they feel like giving up, assuming themselves to be at fault for 'failing'. It's causing a breakdown in trust in what should be a brilliant industry, and I fear that instead of seeking genuine professional help, a lot of people will inevitably seek none.

What can we do?

So yes, the fitness industry is in bad shape. I've been tempted to even say I want nothing to do with it. But I believe that as one of the biggest and most influential industries, we are in a position to make positive change to what is soon going to be the largest cause of preventable death – namely obesity – and we need to begin that change right now.

Rather than turning my back on it all, perhaps going into business coaching where I could charge personal trainers to build their own 'six-figure business' (just like everyone else's), I'm writing this book to try to turn things around for good. For this to happen, I need to dismantle the existing beliefs that hold up some of the most unhelpful and damaging pseudoscience* that's everywhere you look today.

For one thing, the supplement industry continues to mislead consumers as to what they truly need and to mis-sell them many supplements that they don't require; this corner of the industry has its own agenda based on financial gain. Most one-size-fits-all cookie-cutter plans market 'essential' supplementation to bolster their earnings. And in reality, often the most bespoke thing about a plan like this is having your name added to it before it's exported to a PDF file.

Also, personal-trainer (PT) qualifications are not thorough enough, and the fact that many PTs can qualify in just six weeks before finding themselves on the gym floor with little to no experience of working with clients, let alone running a business, means that they often increase their incomes by selling the aforementioned useless

---

* Pseudoscience – 'a collection of beliefs or practices mistakenly regarded as being based on scientific method'.

supplements, and even in some cases join popular pyramid schemes. The majority of PTs also go out of business within their first two years, leaving an exceptionally large churn rate behind them. So the average amount of experience that a modern-day trainer has accrued is often not enough to deal with the complexities of current obesity issues.

The governing bodies of personal training need to look beyond their quick £3,000 transaction fix and, instead, ensure that they are producing trainers who can go out into the industry confidently and correctly. People's health and quality of life are on the line here: remembering eight stretches and memorizing the names of a couple of the bones in the forearm simply won't cut it when a client walks in pre-Type II diabetic, desperate for help to get their health and training on track.

This plays back into that elephant in the room: **all around us people we love are getting sick, health markers are plummeting by the day and obesity is on the rise in adults and children.** Misinformation is rife, but with this book I will change all that, giving you knowledge and tools for life that you can implement independently. Almost immediately you'll begin to change; your attitude, ethos and daily actions will soon have the power to influence those around you – friends, family, loved ones and even colleagues.

Should this pay forward in the way I intend, we can not only turn around the industry, but the lives of those around us. If we all chip in and do our part, we can literally change the world. Think about that every time you see this book; for that reason maybe leave it somewhere in plain sight, like on your pillow or a screenshot of it as your wallpaper on your phone, to remind you each day to continue a little bit further.

Friendly fire

A dietitian can study for bloody years to get qualified, then see a fresh-faced PT in their first year earning double what they are, not to mention the debt from their student loan to become a dietitian. This causes big rifts between two professions that should ideally complement each other, leading to bitter debates across social media and strong divides between the two.

This cannot be blamed on the PT, nor the dietitian; it's just one of many issues we have within an industry that doesn't currently have any regulations or repercussions for spreading misinformation or propaganda that isn't rooted in fact for personal or financial gain.

Here's the thing: I've made a load of mistakes as a personal trainer in my time. Of course I have – I studied for just six weeks to qualify! In hindsight, I can't believe I was allowed on to the gym floor as a professional with so little knowledge. We need to upskill trainers and set a baseline of education for them, so that we're all working from the same page and aiming towards the same goal. This would reduce conflict between trainers and dietitians and generate more positive results.

In addition to the rifts between people who are all on the same team, a lot of what is posted on social media is based more on engagement than education itself. Following and engagement will determine how much someone is worth for a paid post, so it's quite common for people to post a very misleading caption or even to cherry-pick parts of a study to cause a big stir. There are many agendas in all directions, and unfortunately, people kick with the wind when trends arise. And, of course, the last person to benefit is the consumer.

'Fitness events'

If you go to a major fitness expo, expecting to see collaborations from industry icons, mainstream education for trainers and consumers, and examples of what fitness can accomplish, you'll be disappointed. In reality, you'll see none of the aforementioned. What you will see instead is more of a parade.

'Athletes' up to their eyeballs in banned substances, usually anabolic steroids, showing off their anabolic gains – they'll make the expo their peak week; #selfiecentral; stalls on every corner promoting supplements, most of which are not going to benefit the majority of people (supplements to me are like worrying about icing on a cake that's not even been baked yet).

Unfortunately, it doesn't pay well to be in very good shape, despite having hundreds of thousands of followers, sometimes even millions. How do I know? Because if it did, these 'athletes' wouldn't be working for £100 to tense all day on a stand, having to ask for permission to go for a piss. Not only do they get in peak condition for the weekend of the event, they also look very different in the flesh: you can't digitally enhance your appearance in real life, and even the best pair of leggings can't cover the fact that you Photoshopped the majority of your Instagram posts.

You'll walk around and see a plethora of stringer vests, protein-bar samples and businesses promoting the latest fad, whether it be BCAA (see p.210) drinks or exogenous ketones, both relatively useless supplements. Also, from what I've seen, these expos have become more of an arena for narcissists than for fitness people, and it's quite sad to see the rise of anabolic steroid use in recent years. Especially when so many people don't quite know what they're letting themselves in for.

Don't get me wrong, everyone has their poison. For some it's alcohol and partying, for others it's cycling large doses of anabolic steroids. The bodybuilders, more often than not, eat a better diet, focus on sleep and a lot of them lead very healthy lifestyles – my issue isn't with the use of steroids per se; I don't condone it, but I'm not anti either. My issue is to do with the lack of transparency between these bodybuilders and their following, which can be millions of people at a time. Even if we take, conservatively, 50 per cent of the following of an athlete with 2 million followers, that's a million men and women looking up to, and aspiring to look like, this athlete. These people might have less gifted genetics, a different socioeconomic status, full-time jobs with long working hours and they may even have kids. They will buy the athlete's cookie-cutter guide to become 'beach ready in 30 days', then, when they don't see much improvement, they will buy the recommended supplement stack to 'boost' progress. Little do they know they're being misled. The athlete, whether intentionally or not, is skewing the perception of what is accomplishable naturally, and this is a fundamental cause of poor self-esteem, low confidence and a plethora of insecurities, which will affect many aspects of someone's life and, ultimately, their mental health.

Put this on repeat and you'll see the true nature of what fitness has become. It is a playground of dishonesty, narcissism and the pursuit of capital gain. The obese get no closer to a solution, and the ones who are in shape remain depressed, comparing themselves to their idols and getting disheartened with every effort, day after day.

To put it cynically, a disheartened consumer becomes a profitable consumer. The modern-day expo is like flashing a Ferrari at a homeless man, then offering him a lottery ticket: *All this could be yours, as long as you buy a ticket (or a BCAA stack with free shipping).*

Unfortunately, this could not be further from the truth. When I talk about anabolic steroids I'm not just talking about the men, but women too. All prepared to diet and restrict harshly for twenty weeks, often just so they are in 'peak' condition on the supplement stall.

The evidence-based approach to nutrition isn't always sexy, and it certainly isn't favoured by social-media algorithms as much as a bloke with his top off next to a Lamborghini (which he's probably rented for his photoshoot). And should you attend a talk with an evidence-based, qualified speaker you will see:

- a minimal space on the smallest platform with a microphone on the quietest setting, barely audible to the several dozen attendees who are struggling to hear what's being said.
- a small group of personal trainers who actually want to upskill their knowledge (the rest naively thinking they know everything about dealing with people of all shapes and sizes from their six-week PT course).

I'm going to get a bit of hate for saying this, but I will not 'prep' anyone for a bodybuilding or physique show. I think it's pretty poor to represent fitness by starving yourself for twelve to twenty weeks, to cover yourself in fake tan, carb up last minute and force a smile on stage for a row of judges, pretending you're happy when the truth is you're malnourished (so much so that a man loses his libido to the extent that he struggles to get an erection, while a lot of women's menstrual cycles discontinue and their libidos suffer too). I think this is the time for the 95 per cent of competitors who feel this way to take a hint. Your body is trying to tell you something from thousands of years of evolution.

There is a small percentage of bodybuilders that I respect for their work in the competing space, but the misconception that you can't be a decent PT or know much about fat loss unless you have competed is fuelled by those who are less than honest with their real approach, and that concept is completely untrue. I am evidence of that.

The biggest unspoken reason as to why people compete is to create enough external pressure on themselves to ensure that they stick to an over-restrictive diet. Every time they head to the fridge or get hungry, they think about how many people they'll let down if they pull out of the competition. Most hire a 'prep coach', so that they can adhere to the calories set: someone to tell them to go do their sixty minutes of fasted cardio. I think it's damaging to glamourize over-restriction and extreme low body-fat percentages. Unfortunately, many people suffer with eating disorders inside the fitness industry; it's just much easier to hide if they're in good shape. Poor relationships with food exist at both ends of the spectrum, and, from what I've seen, entering your first physique competition is a sure way of developing either a poor relationship with food or your physique – sometimes even both.

There are boutique personal-training franchises that won't hire you as a PT unless you're a certain body-fat percentage, which I also find pathetic. Trying to quantify a coach's ability by their composition is one of the most toxic symptoms at the root of what's wrong with the fitness industry – among everything else, that is.

The thief of joy: why comparison and choice are preventing your progress

Imagine if I told you that you don't need a six-pack to be 'fit', to be accepted, to be loved or to be successful. What if I told you that you could eat pizza and not have to justify it as a 'cheat meal'? What if I told you that you're not inherently bad at dieting or a lost cause, just that you've been intentionally misled into fads and plans that often set you up for inevitable failure?

Although I've pointed out some of the major issues with the industry, I'm not here to completely scare you away from it. In time, it can serve people in the way it should, but something needs to change, and the only way we can do that is first to come to terms with what it really is and then move the goalposts accordingly: as to what is 'fitness' and what is the peak.

In the corporate world, people are living their lives to see who can die with the most money instead of seeking an ultimate work–life balance. We see a similar misconception in fitness, where the goal is to see who can die with the most followers, not how to live a full and balanced life.

I just want to make you aware of what's truly going on behind the picture-perfect Instagram feeds. And it's not only the majority of consumers who are left disheartened by this, but a huge number of new professionals within the industry too. It's all too common for these professionals to compete in physique to fit in with what is now a norm in the industry. 'What's that, James, you haven't competed? What do you know, then? Why should I trust you? Why isn't your profile picture of you on stage?'

Is it really worth giving up 95 per cent of your life for a 5 per cent change in bodyweight?

To me, quite simply: no.

I'd like to think I've accomplished great things in my life so far, and none of them have had anything to do with my physique. I love to be active, I love to train, I feel great when I eat healthily and I feel great when I indulge. I want the same for you, and I'm sure I can help you to feel the same way by the time you've reached the end of this book.

When you understand and absorb what I'm going to teach you here it's going to be incredibly hard for industry charlatans to squeeze any more cash out of you, let alone waste your time.

The industry continues to be far too extreme: from super-restriction and dieting down to unhealthy body-fat percentages, before most of these 'athletes' burn out and go back to old eating habits. After a physique comp, when you step off the stage, you're quite literally primed from a physiological and psychological standpoint for weight gain.

This is particularly relevant to females, who need body fat more than males. It's a rarity to find someone who sits healthily at a very low body-fat percentage without then suffering from a range of other health problems, as you'll find out later in the book (see p.261).

Also, something you're not told is that women who compete often have periods of weeks where they can't sit down for too long as it hurts their tailbone.

However, when they go back to what is a healthy body-fat percentage, they feel a new sensation they didn't before: they feel 'fat'.

Yes, I might sound cynical, but I've seen it happen too many times, and I want to expose the reality behind the myths for you, especially when they have such a negative impact on not just those searching for genuine help, but for the people in the industry who are supposed to be the ones helping too.

To put it in perspective: a teenage girl scrolling through Instagram might double tap that photo, commenting '#bodygoals'. That same teenager would never have been exposed to the sport of 'competing' or seen such lean females if it wasn't for social media. The young girl hasn't even left school and she's already beginning to feel inadequate for having a small amount of body fat. I think the elephant in the room here is that there is a 'sport' out there that has the potential to cause a huge dent in someone's self-esteem, and the sport in this case is competing in physique.

My vision of what a PT should do for their client resembles the relationship between a driving instructor and their pupil. The only real difference is that there is an age limit for driving, but essentially you get to a point in your life when you are legally able to upskill yourself to be proficient behind the wheel of a car on the road. You lack the experience and understanding, so you hire someone on a short-term basis to teach you the fundamentals, so that, in time, you can be good enough to take the wheel on your own without continual help. You learn to become aware of your surroundings, trust your instincts and remain in control. This is what I want to do for you when it comes to your life of dieting, training and day-to-day general no-bullshit nutrition.

Although we may not be the 'finished product' when we pass our driving test, we're in a position where we don't always need someone sitting next to us, making sure that we're doing it right. See where I am going with this? This is where I see a small flaw in PT training across the board, something that made me feel like a bit of a fraud for a long time. Am I the driving instructor who still sits in the car charging an hourly rate, despite my client being able to do it alone? Am I holding back from fully educating my client because I'm so worried about my income shrinking?

Imagine for a second your friend comes to meet you for a coffee, tells you about their third driving instructor in the last couple of years. 'Third?' you'd say. 'What the hell are you paying these people for if they're not teaching you what you require to no longer need them?'

We would very much have an issue with a revolving door of driving instructors, yet in the fitness industry it's a never-ending conveyor belt of new methods to essentially always try to reach the same goal, which looks something like this:

'Hi James, so I did the HIIT plan cooking from scratch, I did the Atkins, I did the low-carb with that woman, I did the high-fat with that man and I did the juicing with that couple. And now I'm here to see what you can do for me.'

I have no problem with industries being profitable. I mean, this is the age of capitalism. However, I do have an issue with the industry titans with an agenda to make millions of pounds, leaving the consumer no better off, and sometimes even worse off than before. We have got to the stage where so many different parties are contradicting each other and promoting their own beliefs (not backed by science) by laying down so many options on the table, that I'm worried there is too much choice. And that out of all the complex and confusing options, for someone whose health is being detrimentally affected by obesity, **they end up choosing none**.

A Brief History of James Smith

The reason many of the topics I will cover in this book will resonate with you on a deep and personal level is because I've made almost all the mistakes a person can make very early on in their career and I think I've adapted fairly well. I did what I thought was right instead of what I wanted, I ended up very unhappy and no longer felt passionate and, even worse, bored. I ballooned in weight in a corporate job I didn't enjoy, and although I felt like I was doing the right thing career-wise, I suddenly became the person drinking on their lunch break to avoid the harsh reality that I didn't like my job, despite how well it paid, and the even harsher reality behind that – that I didn't really like my life either.

We're worried about Brexit, Trump, obesity, cancer, finances and finding true love, but there's one critical disease I was never warned or educated about – a disease that nearly took me down a path of ill health, poor decisions and an uncontrollable urge for a bad diet.

That disease is boredom.

I was neither a very active nor athletic child. I ate too much and exercised infrequently. I have memories from primary school of looking at the food on offer and asking the dinner ladies as I moved down the line, 'Excuse me, Miss, is this fattening?' pointing at every food in turn. No one could really give me a clear answer – no one at school and no one at home. I wasn't sure if it was my fault. Had I missed something? Why were other kids not fat like me? Was it the food I was eating? Was it due to not being in the football team or was it perhaps just something to do with my family tree?

At the age of nine or ten I had nowhere to turn for advice on how to be … less fat. So please realize as you read this that what you are learning goes further than yourself: a cousin, sibling, your own child or a colleague – someone somewhere is confused and you'll have the answer I never had as a child to pass on to them. Although it took fifteen years from that point in the school canteen to taking my first steps in the industry as a PT, the way I felt about how I looked was in my thoughts from a very young age and always at the back of my mind. And I'd be lying if I said it isn't still today.

I spent the majority of primary school in the cloakroom with the special-education kids; teachers were never quite sure what was wrong with me, but I was labelled disruptive by almost all of them. When I was ten, my parents were asked to give me music to listen to in class so that I wouldn't disrupt the other kids.

Six years later, I was asked politely to 'leave school'. So my mum took me to the Jobcentre, smashed my Nokia 3310 in the road as we left school (a physical feat in itself) and told me not to come home without a job. But instead, in a bid to dodge that annoying thing you do as an adult, commonly known as 'employment', I enrolled in the BTEC course at a sports college. And so began my passion for fitness and sport.

I then began a journey of actually enjoying the learning process. I studied for four more years on a sports studies course before trying my hand at the fully fledged university BSc, but it wasn't long before getting drunk each night won the battle over attending lectures, and at twenty-one, I ventured into the 'real world' without a formal degree.

> *'The opposite of love is indifference, and the opposite of happiness is boredom.'*
>
> Timothy Ferriss, *The 4-Hour Workweek*

Almost a decade later, I can remember four or five separate occasions I'd consider to be mini mid-life crises and that each and every one was absolutely fucking fantastic, because I have loved and embraced the changes that resulted from them. Change is something humans inherently dislike, but which, unfortunately, the large majority of us need.

At twenty-four, I was working in finance recruitment, doing what was considered 'the right thing to do': being paid well at a nine-to-five with good 'career opportunities', while having to conform to being clean-shaven in a flipping suit and being asked by everyone, 'How was your weekend?' And the funny thing is that although I'm an open person, I was not honest once. I think two of us out of nearly thirty were not married, and the last thing they would have wanted to hear was how, in fact, I'd necked a bottle of wine on a rugby bus in my underpants.

Every few hours of every single day I was going to make coffee, quite simply out of boredom to get myself away from my desk where I sat surrounded by people who could handle the level of boredom that came with the role. I'd be productive enough to seem busy, but the truth is I was bored. So fucking bored. People never give credit to how exhausting it is to pretend to be busy. It's soul destroying.

All for what? A rat race. To see who can die with the most money.

Looking back at the quite ridiculous weekends that made up nearly a third of my life I can only see it as a form of escapism from the dreary existence of working in a job I didn't have any passion for. Was it any wonder I turned to getting wasted most weekends? Although I admittedly still enjoy a fun weekend, I'd say, hand on heart, that the reasons behind these indulgences *now* come from a positive place. But it's only in hindsight that I can see that.

By being dubbed the 'Calorie Fucking Deficit' guy I've come to realize many of our 'vices', whether alcohol or calorie-dense foods, are a crutch to help us through low periods, or a form of escapism, masquerading as an innocent pleasure or a 'treat'. This narrative of quite simply 'eating too much', 'being greedy' or even 'lazy' is also quite naive; it goes much deeper than that – the cause of modern-day obesity, that is – and we'll be getting into that in more detail as we go on.

One of my crises eventually led to me backpacking in Southeast Asia, and when you find out how much of a good time you can have living off just £15 a day, your perspective changes pretty quickly. However, six months in, I began to realize how hard it is to have a work–life balance when you don't have any work. So, back on UK soil, I became a personal trainer in 2014 and moved back in with my parents,* six years before publishing this book.

People often ask me, 'If you were not a PT what would you do instead?' And in response, I find myself with a mental blank, because I'm really not sure. To me, I've reached the peak. My passion is fitness, sport and coaching people, and this is what I do every day. I've been on a tremendous journey from a confused fat kid with learning difficulties to a published author, credited as a respected expert in his field of fat loss and coaching. Any success credited to me in my professional life can only come off the back of **having eventually aligned my passion with my daily life and career, and most of all, being happy with what I choose to do every day**.

Eating better and exercising frequently are not chores to me, not a part of what I *need* to do. I genuinely enjoy every aspect of it because I enjoy my life. I am no longer bored because I love my work. There's

* No matter what journey you're on, ask yourself: if you take a risk, a huge risk, something that could change your life for the better, what truly is the worst circumstance on the flip side? Moving in with your parents again? I did it in the middle of my twenties, and I tell you what: it's a lot easier to go after your ambitions with two hands – especially if you're lucky enough to have parents like mine.

always something you can do to occupy you when your work aligns with your passion.

I'm still a fat kid at heart. I love crisps and dips, ordering several entrées and nothing better than slouching into bed come 9 p.m. And some days, I don't even set an alarm to wake up.

I am the same as you, I promise. I have maybe just learned the tools I need to adapt certain aspects of my life to create better balance, which brings me on to the rest of the book: not only will I educate you on fat loss and training, but first I will help you to address the factors that go beyond fitness and diet that are currently holding you back from achieving your goals. We all need foundations to build on, and the next deep and powerful part of this book is about to begin.

Why is it that you're fatter than you'd like to be?

Consumer – Method – Principle

For a moment I want you to imagine that you are the **consumer** (on the left) and, irrespective of your goal, right in front of you are a load of **methods** – the industry's way of dressing up what you will need to put into practice. There are methods all over the place, all confusing and contradicting, and each proclaiming to be the 'ultimate' way to accomplish your **goal i.e. fat loss**.

The **principle** sits on the far side (on the right); you can't quite see it yet as dozens of methods are in the way. You can see so many of these methods that have been forced upon you over the years, and little did you know that on the other side of them sits one common element on its own: that singularity is the principle.

The principle when it comes to fat loss is a calorie deficit.

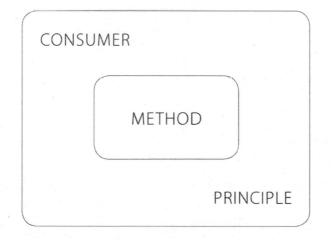

This is the only way we can successfully lose fat. I'll get into the details of what exactly calorie deficit means shortly, but for now, imagine you on the left and what you desperately need on the right.

The method is how you package the principle for the consumer.

For too long, the method has kept the consumer at arm's length from what they actually need to know and do in order to change their body and their health status for the better. We've seen the principle hidden among the 'diets' below, which, for our purposes, we will call the 'methods'.

A brief explanation of popular methods

The following are just a few of the mainstream methods used for creating a calorie deficit.

The 5:2 diet

Imagine, if you will, that you have a slight spending problem. You then decide to leave your credit card at home for two days of the week. You notice a decrease in spending week on week, and so this is your chosen method for spending less money. In essence, this is how the 5:2 diet works: the consumer restricts calories fairly aggressively for two days of the week, which brings down the week's total calorie intake.

I very rarely advocate this for my clients except in some circumstances, which I will go into in more detail later in the book. I prefer the 2:5 diet, where I eat less Monday to Friday and then indulge at the weekend. The 5:2 diet becomes a little more altered (and often complicated) each time someone puts their own spin on how it is done, which changes the approach and risks the effectiveness and understanding of the principle of the diet itself.

The ketogenic diet

When we look at the foods we eat, they can be subdivided into cate-gories known as 'macros', which is short for 'macronutrients'. When I first saw this word, I thought to myself, This lingo isn't for me – it's five syllables and sounds bloody complex. I will explain macros a bit more in later chapters (see p.78), but for the time being, let me categorize a few foods into the relevant groups for you:

Protein

Protein is a macronutrient, obtained from foods like chicken, fish and some dairy products, such as whey protein, cheese, yoghurt.

Carbohydrates

These include things like rice, bread, fruits and vegetables.*

Carbohydrates are broken down into sugar (glucose) when digested. This means that anything that consists primarily of sugar – for instance sweets, desserts, etc. – is also labelled a carbohydrate. Now, carbohydrates are not inherently bad for us. On the contrary – they are our bodies' preferred source of energy. However, when a 'low-carb zealot' preaches propaganda about the life-threatening effects of eating carbs, you obediently eradicate them, only to realize that you've removed a rather large number of foods from your diet. And, remember, that food (*any* food) equals calories. Pasta, bread, sandwiches, cake, desserts, biscuits, dairy, sweets, fizzy drinks, alcohol … I could go on. Eradicating a plethora of foods like this from anyone's diet will, of course, create a substantial calorie deficit. This

---

* Dietary fats, which make up the large part of calories in this diet, are another significant food group to mention, and are found in things like eggs, cooking oils and avocado.

will lead to fat loss, but it is all too often simplistically and anecdotally attributed to the benefits of being on a 'low-carb' diet.

If you removed one-third of macronutrients, I'm not surprised you lost body fat, to be honest, mate.

A state of ketosis is where you limit carbohydrates (or calories) to such an extent that the amount of sugar (glucose) in the blood becomes so low that it has to react accordingly, and the body then produces a similar source of energy called 'ketones' from fat (consumed and stored). When the amount of ketones in the blood reaches a certain level, we are said to be in a state of ketosis. Often, people believe they're in a state of ketosis, but really, they're just low carb. I'll expand a little later in the book (see p.232) on the rare occasions I may promote this diet for some populations; however, across the board, with the intention of finding a sustainable diet that is easy to maintain over long periods of time, I think it's important that we consider other options when looking to create a deficit – a better 'method', so to speak – and one that allows for flexibility.

Vegetables and fruit also sit within the category of carbohydrates – all fibre, starches and sugars to be precise.

Most people who adhere to a ketogenic diet believe it has superior fat loss over any other diet. To this day, however, I have not seen any literature to back that claim.

16:8/Intermittent Fasting (IF)

Wow, aren't millennials great? They took 'skipping breakfast' and made it 'intermittent fasting'.

The usual protocol within this method is to refrain from your first feeding until 1 p.m., after which you're allocated eight hours in which to consume food, then after 9 p.m. you have to discontinue it until the following day. Again, a lot of anecdotal claims are held up against intermittent fasting, and I'll delve into them later in the book (see p.246); however, it's always simply a case of 'skipping a meal, mate'. And if you remove one in three major meals of the day, that's seven fewer meals a week, 365 fewer meals a year – which, for someone who consumes 700 calories per meal, is 255,500 calories per year, equating to approximately 73 lb of fat.

As with many methodologies, the person or brand promoting it will claim that theirs is superior to any other, especially when challenged. I sit in the camp of personal preference and, as I'll explain a little later, the science says there aren't tangible benefits to fat loss in shortened feeding windows vs total caloric restriction (comparable to managing your daily spending vs shortening the windows in which you spend).

These methods can annoy me because often the consumer is left in the dark about the principle – not only that but they're sold with a pinch of pseudoscience. Every method for fat loss is often touted to have benefits to reduce cancer, and I wouldn't be surprised if, within the year, someone says intermittent fasting makes you taller. People are getting distracted from why they picked the protocol in the first place. Can skipping breakfast help you lose fat? Yes. What if you fancy eating breakfast? Then eat it. Just don't become sidetracked by what's being preached by someone who's declared themselves a professional in breakfast skipping at the expense of finding a method that actually works for you.

The low-fat diet

When looking at macronutrients, which I will do in more detail later (see p.79), technically, per gram, protein and carbohydrates have the same amount of calories (4kcals), while dietary fats have 9 calories per gram; this is two-and-a-quarter times as many as proteins and carbs. This led to an era – especially around the 1990s – when people tried to remove as much fat from their diets as possible, and many foods were labelled 'low fat' to lure the consumer into purchasing without guilt.

We need a certain amount of our daily energy intake to come from dietary fats – around 20 per cent is the ball-park figure I like to work with. Less than this can be detrimental to our production of essential hormones, which we need in order for our bodies to feel, look and perform at their best. So it's very important that at no point do we allow our intake of dietary fats to fall below that amount.

Popular slimming clubs and weight-tracking organizations

I'm not going to delve into these too much, but it's quite apparent that they have their own agendas, where they purposely avoid talking about calories or calorie counting, but they still endorse it (for profit) by giving it their own terms. The easiest way to know this is when these organizations bring out their own brand of biscuits, ready meals or even shakes on which the small print says, 'Must be consumed as part of a calorie-controlled diet.' This is a legal disclaimer that forces them to confess to the importance of calorie control irrespective of whether their system directly refers to it.

My approach

I have been training clients since 2014. I have several-thousand hours of coaching experience on the gym floor, working with all kinds of people, and I believe that a huge component of the education necessary to become a good coach needs to happen right there. I'm not saying my approach is perfect – it's not a magic pill, and I need you to put in as much as I do to get anything out of it – but it is working for a lot of my clients, as well as those who follow me on social media. I'll share a bit more about my methods here.

I have intentionally cultivated a following, not only to give people a new way of thinking or a new perspective on elements of their journey towards improving fitness and health, but also to cut out the bullshit, which I come across each and every day. But I don't just want to make noise on my own – I want you to join me. Don't stand for misinformation and don't let your friends, family and other people you know be misled.

So yes, I'm an intentional disruptor at the same time as an educator, but **one of the main goals of my work is to put the consumer 'in bed' with the principle, so you can fully understand how sustainable and long-term fat loss occurs**. And I want to do this so that companies profiting from your confusion, frustration and repeat business will no longer be able to keep you so far away from the only bit of information you'll ever actually need if you are to successfully and sustainably lose weight and feel better. That's not to mention having better confidence and self-esteem, shagging with the lights on, wearing colours other than black, going running in just a sports bra (or topless, for men – unless you're a bloke who is into wearing sports bras, that is).

Imagine for a moment that you are the frog in this scenario:

If you put a frog in hot water it will jump out; however, if you put a frog in cold water and heat it slowly, it'll happily boil to death.

I don't want to put you in an environment that you want to jump out of straight away. I want you to be comfortable and not think about jumping every time I turn the heat up. I think of this whenever I consider implementing any kind of lifestyle change with clients. I'd like to think that over the years, I've become experienced at finding ways to make change for each client's needs, rather than reinventing the wheel every time I make an alteration to someone's diet or training regime.

It would be very easy for me to bunch some workouts and recipes together and flog the same thing to everyone. I could even write a cookbook – pay a chef to write it and slap my face on the front. Not only that, but I could even put a supplement discount code in there too, so that I get a kickback on every transaction. However, that's not how I want to conduct my business. I am an educator, a coach, and I want to spread the good word like a modern-day Messiah (but with better banter!).

I'm going to assume that right now, you are where I have been before. I know how it feels and how frustrating it is. I know what it's like to wake up and consider throwing in the towel on your lifestyle idealism and ambitions for your physique.

To me, you're not just a reader; you're not a prospect; you're not a consumer; you're not a transaction or a way for me to make it rain with cash during my time in the limelight. To me, you're a real person and I'm going to make sure that you are no longer victim to, or a part of, someone else's agenda to make money. My main objective for my time in this industry is to make the principle – the only one you actually need to do well – feel like second nature to you. Once you're in bed with it, so to speak, it will liberate not only you, but those around you too.

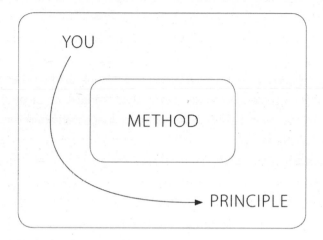

Fat loss vs muscle gain

I'm going to assume the large majority of readers would like to lose fat. I know many of you want to build muscle too, but seeing as obesity is a worldwide epidemic, I will start with fat loss. It's also worth noting that many of us who say we want to 'lose fat and build muscle' already have a considerable amount of muscle, it's just not visible yet. And for anyone who is not sure whether to build muscle or lose fat, my advice is to lose fat first. Ideally, you should get lean, then look to build muscle. I will go into a little more detail, for those interested, below and in Part 2.

Some of you are already in great shape and would tell me, 'James, I want to lose fat.' If you were my face-to-face client, I'd kick you in the shins because you don't need to. You need to fall in love with your training and set some performance goals – you're just a bit lost with your goal setting, that's all. Too many people want to go from great shape to very great shape, purely based on what they're exposed to on social media. I want those people to be paired up with a challenging performance goal instead of starving themselves for a new profile picture.

If you have the opportunity, please at least try to fall in love with the pursuit of a performance goal rather than the unfulfilling pursuit of looking your 'best'. I don't think that a lot of people fully understand the implications of fat and weight loss; when people ask me about what goal they should aim for despite carrying around a fair amount of excess weight, I say this: 'Okay, let's begin with fat loss,' because the reality is that once a certain amount of fat has been lost, there's a lot more muscle already there than people realize. To put it in perspective, 1 litre of water weighs 1 kilogram. So let's imagine you're hosting a dinner party and you realize you need some mixers: you nip down to the local store and grab a 2 litre bottle of tonic water, then decide you actually need three. As you pay, the person at the checkout asks if you would like a bag. For that amount, you may even need to double bag for the ten-minute walk home. I want you to think about how heavy that bag will be with three 2 litre bottles of tonic water in it …

The point of this analogy is that 6 kilograms can feel like a lot, but in the world of fat loss it is not actually difficult for someone to lose that amount of weight. When looking to improve someone's performance in a given sport, we tend to look at all the complex things first, but usually being less fat – and therefore lighter – is a huge benefit that is often overlooked. So imagine hugging those three bottles close to your chest and going for a run, then walking up several flights of stairs. Imagine how you'd feel putting the shopping bags down and then repeating all of that without them – you'd feel ten years younger and move around like a spring chicken.

So I hope you're starting to see that fat and weight loss aren't just about your next Instagram picture on holiday. They are about being able to keep up with your kids in the park, seeing that an elevator is full and being happy to walk up two flights of stairs instead, or improving your footwork to trick your savvy dog when throwing a tennis ball in the park.

How to build muscle effectively will be covered briefly in the book; **resistance training has a plethora of benefits for bone health, muscles and general health, yes. But losing fat – losing the weight – has to be the priority for most**. Muscle is tissue that shortens when contracted to create locomotion. Body fat, especially too much, quite literally increases the chances of developing serious chronic diseases, endangering not only physical health, but mental health as well.

I am going to empower, enable and educate you – and through you, your friends, your family members and your colleagues too – so you can seasonally get 'fat' from time to time without feeling like a failure. Yeah, that's right. I want you to get a bit fat: on holiday, at Christmas and when you next go through a slight flat period with your training – because gaining fat is cyclical and a normal part of being a regular human. The problems begin with not knowing how to lose that fat, and when you learn how to do that your life will become less stressful. **Food will taste great without bringing feelings of guilt or shame, and you will feel empowered to make decisions**, not only about your diet and fitness, but also your social life and attitude towards your own body. You'll plan meals better, improve drink choices and not beat yourself up for enjoying yourself.

What if you get injured? I want you to be mentally prepared for that too. Shit happens and you need to know you will gain weight when you're injured. But as I said, gaining weight is only an issue when you don't know how to lose it.

We also need to look at things like periods near Christmas. I've put clients in a controlled surplus before, as I'd rather they adhered to twice their maintenance* than just going crazy and consuming everything that's put in front of them. Giving yourself something to stick to makes you feel a lot better.

I'm not sure what you're doing next Christmas but I'll be getting festively plump.

If I was here as your financial advisor, and said either, 'Right, let's put 50 per cent of everything you earn away and not touch it,' or, 'Look, I want you to put 10 per cent away every day; it's going to take five times longer than the previous approach, but the good news is it'll hardly feel like you're even saving money,' you'd probably be sensible and pick the latter, right? Sometimes taking things out of context can bring clarity to these situations.

Over the next few-thousand wonderful words I'll not only be talking about fitness, but also explaining to you some laws that exist in our universe and inside our minds, holding us back, making us misinterpret our surroundings and situations, so that ultimately you can implement the necessary changes to improve your life. Why? *Because it's all a part of my approach.*

So let's get into it …

---

* Maintenance is how many calories you require in a day in order to maintain your weight and size. Sometimes giving someone twice their maintenance could still mean a reduction in caloric intake vs not tracked.

The Calorie Deficit

calorie*

'The energy needed to raise the temperature of 1 gram of water through 1°C.'

deficit

'The amount by which something is too small.'

Calorie deficit, also known as an energy deficit, is a term that you may or may not have heard before. It is the scientific equation that is required for human beings to lose body fat. **It is, in fact, the principle behind every fat-loss diet in history.**

Question:

How does [insert any common diet] work for fat loss?

Answer:

Calorie Deficit.

* Some smartarse at some point will want to differentiate a calorie from a kcal – for the purposes of this book, all calorie mentions refer to kcals (kilocalories). A banana that contains 100 kcals technically contains 100,000 calories, but this book is not about comparing penis sizes, so let's carry on.

Here's how I explain this when I first meet a client: let's say that after a few years, you have successfully saved some money in your current account, and let's say that the more money you have saved, the more fat you have on your body. If you have excess funds or 'savings' in your bank account, then you have retained more money than you have spent. Translating that into a caloric intake and body-fat context, this means you have eaten more calories (in) than you have expended through daily life and exercise (out).

If you were trying to ensure that you were saving more than you spent, you'd be pretty pissed off when you checked your bank balance and saw it at £0.00. So how can we expect any different when this is translated into an energy consumption and expenditure context? This is where the zealots mentioned earlier come in, with misleading advice on why you haven't lost any fat – maybe you didn't drink enough of the right kind of tea, or take the right supplements, or eat your meals at the right time of day, let alone cook the right foods for your 'body type'? **However, it is, in almost every case a simple miscalculation (whether intentional or not) of energy in vs energy out.**

So when intending to lose fat successfully, we need to do the opposite of what a smart financial advisor would suggest. We need to tilt the balance to transition into burning more than we spend. This can be done through earning less (consuming fewer calories) or spending more (burning more through exercise) – it's up to the person in question, but usually a sensible amount of both is optimal.

We don't have to be in a deficit every day. Think of finances again: let's say you're getting paid at the end of every weekday. You save 15 per cent of the money you get paid each day, but at weekends you decide to spend one day's 15 per cent on having a good time. You're still saving in that scenario: one day off from saving doesn't negate your savings; it just creates a slight dent in the long run to the duration of a diet. The less consistent you are, quite simply the longer it will take. How this affects the long-term results varies in each individual case.

There are two types of people in the world: those who occasionally 'fall off the wagon' when dieting, and those who lie about it.

I saw a great post by Sohee Lee, a friend and industry peer, who said, 'When you get a flat tyre, you pull over, but you don't slash the other three tyres for no reason.' This perfectly summarizes what people tend to do when they hit a speed bump in dieting: they give up, throw in the towel and grab the nearest tub of ice cream. But I want you to think about it this way: if you've ever seen something that you can't sensibly afford, but you bought it anyway, you don't then allow yourself to spiral into endless debt and move back in with your parents; you strategically plan around repaying the debt from the purchase and maybe cutting back elsewhere for a limited time period.

The calorie deficit has been dressed up and packaged so many times now through the 'next biggest diet', meal-replacement system or 'secret weight-loss supplement' that it's become almost unrecognizable. In response to my bid to cut through the terminology for the mainstream (along with pent-up emotions), I have been dubbed the 'Calorie Fucking Deficit' guy. If you search on social media for #CFD, that's what it stands for. People wave it as a flag of liberation, as they now understand a principle they once did not.

All low-carb movements, high-fat movements, fasting movements lead back to the calorie deficit. Multimillion-pound slimming clubs even create their own languages, using terms such as 'syns'; it's easy to connect the dots to believe that it's to make the consumer's life easier, but I disagree wholeheartedly.

It's important at this stage to recognize that implementing a calorie deficit is not always straightforward, and usually the bigger it is, the more the body will try to adapt to prevent it from happening. Imagine you have a child, and you find out that they've started spending the savings that you wanted them to have for when they are older. You'd probably step in to ensure they at least slow down, but ideally, you would stop them altogether. Similarly, biology dictates that we have a myriad processes to make fat loss harder.

Human beings have been around for hundreds of thousands of years, and for the majority of our history, we've had to work very hard from one meal to the next – it was a matter of survival of the fittest. Now, when we diet, we are choosing to engage in small periods of starving ourselves, and ideally, we should do it slowly to manage the symptoms of hunger, fatigue, being irritable and poorer performance. Appetite is a part of evolution, and one of the first frontiers to prevent us from losing too much fat too fast.

With that in mind, now is a better time than any to talk about our two main 'hunger hormones': leptin and ghrelin.

For many of you, these may be words you have never heard before, but please keep in mind that I would not have put them in the book unless they were crucial to your understanding of fat loss and your body.

Leptin and ghrelin are the big players in regulating appetite, which consequently influences bodyweight and how much fat we will have 'on us' at any given moment in time.

Similar to a car alerting you when the fuel is too low, ghrelin plays a signalling role, telling you to eat, so you're not too low in fuel reserves or energy. Leptin is similar to that click you hear when you fill up the tank, letting you know that you're full and there's no need to add more fuel. This is to oversimplify other biological roles of leptin, but we don't need to go that far down the rabbit hole.

Although both leptin and ghrelin are secreted in other parts of the body, they both affect our brains.

Leptin is secreted primarily in fat cells, as well as the stomach, heart and skeletal muscle. One of its best-known roles is to decrease hunger.

Ghrelin is secreted primarily in the lining of the stomach, and increases hunger. I usually think of ghrelin sounding like gremlin; if you search for the dictionary definition of a gremlin, you 'll find *'an imaginary mischievous sprite regarded as responsible for an unexplained mechanical or electronic problem or fault'*. That sounds about right.

Both leptin and ghrelin respond to how well fed you are; leptin usually also correlates to fat mass – the more fat you have, the more leptin you produce.

I wanted to name these two hormones because they are related to calories and energy balance, and you'll find their influence in the sleep part of the book really helpful (see p.90). Here's an explanation that revolutionized dieting for me: our response to ghrelin production, aka hunger, is not pleasant; it is, in fact, hundreds of thousands of years of evolution teaching your brain to eat. However, it is cyclical.

Do you know what happens if you endure a bit of hunger for forty-five minutes to an hour? **Nothing.** It goes away almost completely until your next regular feeding window. So next time you're hungry, don't eat, but give yourself an hour to test this theory. Hunger doesn't last for ever; you probably already know that because last time you were genuinely too busy to eat, you forgot all about it and may well have had a surprising moment later on and said, 'I'm not even hungry any more.' That, my friend, was a cyclical bout of ghrelin that came and then went away.

Those who dispute the Calorie Deficit and an introduction to Confirmation Bias

It doesn't take very long to peruse the Internet and find someone with a 'clickbait' title of 'calories in, calories out doesn't work'. This is also spoken about as 'CICO'. When talking about a calorie as a measure of energy *a calorie is always a calorie*.

But are all calories the same? Absolutely not. The body will treat different sources of food differently, whether it's fish, potato, nuts or even chocolate. A hundred kcals of potato will be absorbed differently to the same amount of chicken. The potato, once broken down, may refuel muscles that have just been trained, while the chicken is broken down into amino acids to repair the same muscles. Different roles, same calorie values. So note that although there are complex differentiations between foods, fat loss is still always governed by calories in vs calories out, whether you'd think so or not.

One of the biggest debates fuelled by some of the modern-day morons is that calories don't matter and carbohydrates alone are the issue. There is a hormone you may have heard of before called insulin, which is known as a *storage hormone*. Because of this there are those who hold by what has been named by some of my peers and mentors as the 'insulin hypothesis', which claims that as long as you keep your insulin low, *you will lose fat*.

One nutritionist for a large functional training organization made a sweeping statement to tens of thousands of members, saying: 'The key to fat loss is to manage your insulin.' This is like saying the key to saving money is to manage what items you buy, rather than addressing the total amount being spent vs saved.

Just because a million people say something stupid, that doesn't mean it's not still stupid.

One of the biggest issues I find across the entire industry is this notion of 'association being causation', when the correct way of thinking is to always know that '**association is NOT causation**'. There is a common mentality of connecting dots without logic and often without evidence. For instance, if I observe the M25 motorway in the UK and I see every car crash that takes place, I would note that in fatal car crashes that occur there is often an ambulance on the scene. I could then come to the conclusion that if an ambulance turns up to the scene of an incident, then it is likely to result in a fatal outcome, whereas if no ambulance arrives, it is likely that the incident is less serious. But does this mean that it is because the ambulance is present that the outcome is worse? No, of course not; ambulances are called due to the severity of the incident and can't be drawn in as a factor in fatalities.

It's not always idiots who dispute CICO, though. There are some brilliant minds in the nutrition industry who have accomplished stellar work within the fields of hydration and sports performance, but when it comes to fat loss, they let anecdotal beliefs shroud what the data actually says.

Often people sit in their own camp of what's worked for them, whether that's fasting protocols, low-carb or ketogenic diets – and these diets *do* work for some, but they're not inherently superior to any other protocol outside of a very few medical conditions, such as some forms of epilepsy; however, at this moment in time I haven't seen anything solid in research yet to conclude that.

Unfortunately, when people come across new evidence confirming their existing belief they will trust it. However, if it doesn't agree with their existing belief or understanding, they'll disregard it. People can then cherry-pick the parts of studies that back their own beliefs and dismiss the rest. This is known as the confirmation bias.

People are prone to believe what they want to believe. This is why when I write about certain topics, I will often search for data to prove me wrong rather than right to ensure I have understood both sides of the debate. If you listen to the arguments from low-carb or keto zealots, much of their information is not factual but anecdotal. They say, 'My clients did this,' or, 'I found that this happened when I did that.' I'm not saying that their clients didn't lose fat or accomplish great things, but they're allowing their pre-existing 'carbs are bad' belief to feed their bias. Any new evidence that comes up to oppose this is disregarded and wiped off the table.

I'm not stating that removing some carbohydrates is bad; I'm not saying it doesn't work. It often does (through creating a deficit). A lot of the misinformation isn't malice. But people – and I mean friends, family and colleagues, not just experts – have all been feeding their confirmation bias and now they're trying to feed yours (pardon the pun).

Confirmation bias in action: carbs, protein and insulin

From a pragmatic, personal point of view, I'd like to inform you that insulin is not 'bad', nor does it need to be 'managed' (except in Type I and some Type II diabetics). We secrete small amounts of insulin all the time; if we didn't, we'd be in a lot of trouble. We will talk about diabetes later in the book (see p.111), but for now, when a Type I diabetic increases their protein intake, we can see stabilizations in their blood-sugar levels. This, in turn, means that there is a less frequent requirement for the Type I diabetic to eat foods to raise their blood sugar, therefore making it easier to create or adhere to a calorie deficit. The benefits can be attributed to the fact that protein can help in stabilizing blood sugar. However, if I was to waft that past a low-carb zealot, they'd be the first to point out that the *carbohydrates were to blame*, which is simply too reductive.

Another thing that you should note and bring up in an argument is this: I used to believe that too many carbohydrates would mean that the glucose (sugar) in the blood would then be stored as body fat, because it made complete sense hypothetically. But here's what really happens: the pathway for converting dietary carbohydrate into fat, or de novo lipogenesis (DNL), is present in humans, whereas the capacity to convert fats into carbohydrate does not exist. Now, this process actually rarely occurs. Should you consume the maintenance or deficit calories it is incredibly unlikely that any carbohydrates will be converted into fat. Not only that, but even in a surplus due to the inefficiency of converting carbohydrates into fat, **usually it's the fats from the diet that are stored instead as adipose tissue (body fat).**

Even in overfeeding studies trying to identify any benefits from manipulating high carb or high fat, there seems to be no real quantifiable difference, and all roads seem to lead to the fact that we should be promoting higher amounts of protein rather than lower amounts of carbs:

According to research: 'There appears to be no meaningful difference between overfeeding on a high-carbohydrate or high-fat diet.' The study goes on: 'Dietary protein appears to have a protective effect against fat gain during times of energy surplus, especially when combined with resistance training. Therefore, the evidence suggests that dietary protein may be the key macronutrient in terms of promoting positive changes in body composition.' (See References, p.285.)

Other factors that feed the confirmation bias:

Water weight: when we look at a diet that includes carbohydrates, we need to think about water weight. Carbohydrates are stored for use in muscle tissue (this is known as glycogen) and for every 1 g of carbohydrate that enters a cell, 3–5 g of water usually accompany it. So if you eat 100 g of carbohydrates (400 kcals worth) you could gain 0.3–0.5 kg of water just stored alongside carbohydrates in muscle tissue. On the flip side, we need to consider that most of the weight loss occurring with low-carb diets, especially in the early stages, is water and not fat.

Eradication: when you say to someone with very little nutritional knowledge to eat 'no carbs' they'll tend to know what it means: no bread, pasta, cake, biscuits, alcohol, fizzy drinks, etc. This in itself causes a calorie deficit most of the time. Telling someone to create a deficit tends to be quite nuanced, though, and doesn't always lead to a reduction in calories.

Another important thing to do is to stay away from Netflix documentaries – Netflix is there to entertain, not educate. It's almost as if I need to tell you that *Stranger Things* and *Breaking Bad* are also fiction.

To conclude, everyone in the world will seek to confirm their own beliefs and disregard any that go against them. Be pragmatic with every decision you make, and when asking someone to prove the point behind a thesis or theory, listen out for anecdote – chances are they've been feeding their own confirmation bias with someone else's. It's human nature.

Calorie calculators

Starting points are important, and for a long time as a PT I would ask clients to track their food for a few weeks. I'd then review their intake and make changes. It was a very long-winded process, partly because it's not hugely motivating for a client to ask them to put effort in and not see any short-term returns. In recent years, I have implemented the use of a calorie calculator as a starting point for determining calories.*

There are several different formulas to try to determine how many calories someone needs per day. I use one called the Harris-Benedict, to which I've made some small adjustments. The questionnaire tries to determine your weight, height and age; with that you can get a rough idea of your sedentary expenditure. You're then asked how active you are, and this number is multiplied by a corresponding amount. For instance, 'lightly active' would be the calculated amount x 1.2.

There are some holes you can pick in the accuracy of this approach, but personally, from day one, I think it's imperative to have a tangible goal to aim for. Most people go, 'Wow, my calories look really high.' But comparing them to their excessive indulging at the weekend, they're actually not. Even with a moderate amount of calories, say, 2,000 a day for a female, that's 14,000 a week, and should you want to 'save' some calories in order to have a few drinks and a takeaway over the weekend, then you're left with a fraction of the original figure to play with on weekdays, if you are to stick to the overall target.

Tracking your calories weekly or daily is your prerogative, like balancing your books between payslips with an agenda to save money. As long as you do it, I am not too bothered about how it's micromanaged.

* To use my calorie calculator head to www.jamessmithacademy.com/calculator.

If your calories given from the calculator are **too low**, you'll: (deficit)

- feel very hungry all the time
- be irritable, moody, have brain fog
- experience poor performance, poor recovery, soreness

If your calories are **too high**, you'll notice: (surplus)

- a strange love for your diet
- good moods, good performance
- slow weight gain

If your calories are neither, not a lot will happen. This is known as *maintenance*.

I have said to my clients over the years that the only person who truly knows how those calories will work is the person implementing them. It is for the dieter to find out. Most athletes and fitness professionals roughly know their caloric intake for maintenance and fat loss. They know their 'sweet spot' through playing with their calorie intake almost on a trial-and-error basis. **You need to learn how to do the same – and I am going to help you.**

Protein, as we discussed earlier, is a big player in fat loss and muscle growth too, so my calculator gives a protein goal and a calorie goal. Should you want fat loss, I set a deficit of 15 per cent, which is considered conservative by others in the industry. Should a surplus be required, where someone is looking to optimize muscle growth or weight gain, it's +15 per cent, and maintenance is sticking closely to the proposed figure.

You'll see later in the book about protein targets (p.211), but I set mine at 1.5 g per kilogram. This is conservative too, but a lot of my clientele are new to protein targets and I don't want to throw them in at the deep end too early (or hot water that they'll jump out of).

Macro and calorie calculators are not gospel.

They are, however, a starting point – an essential one – and although their efficacy, early doors, may not be where you'd like it to be, you're the only one in the world who can really dial in what your numbers are. It's worth noting, especially for any of you ladies with Polycystic Ovary Syndrome (PCOS), which you'll come to understand a bit more about later in the book (see p.269), that your targets may differ a lot from the original calculations.

MyFitnessPal (MFP)

This is the app I use to track and log calories. However, I don't get my clients to determine their calories this way. Firstly, MFP asks you how much fat you'd like to lose a week: I don't know anyone who doesn't select the highest option possible, which is 2lb (0.9 kg). A hypothesized 7,000 calorie deficit a week is needed to accomplish that, so people are often left with 1,200 calories, as the app isn't allowed to go any lower, and a lot of people will not sustain their diet on such a large deficit.

Also, MFP gives you the option to 'eat back' calories from exercise, which I don't think should be the case. In essence, this means that there is an amount of ticking calories that increase as you are active throughout the day – as if to say, well, as you moved a lot, you can have more calories; if you're sedentary, you're not allocated the extra calories.

Firstly, you're not a dog who gets rewarded for exercising, and secondly, if you use my calculator, your exercise is already included for each day's calories. Should you miss the gym, I'm sure you'll still be in a deficit, just a smaller one – nothing to cry about.

Why a 'Calorie Fucking Deficit' is more than just a deficit

Self-esteem, confidence and sex drives are plummeting. Social media is driving inadequacies up, people are feeling worse about themselves than ever, mental-health disorders are skyrocketing and we can no longer look at an energy deficit purely as just a mathematical equation of energy in vs energy out.

I've often said that **having fat isn't being fat; being fat is when your composition steals from you each day**, whether it's self-esteem, confidence or even the ability to tell someone you're interested in asking them out without being judged on how overweight you currently are.

So this isn't just a calorie deficit. It's not just about having less fat. This is about feeling completely different and becoming a new person – maybe someone you used to be or someone you have spent your entire life wanting to be. It's about making clear the only concept people need after a history of frustration and unsustainable dieting. It's about how the principle has been intentionally kept out of reach for the people who need it (see p.33).

This isn't new science. It's been known for a long time. People have needed this information desperately, and instead they got sold a recipe book touting how to cook from scratch or the idealism of intuitive eating, as if that was the real hidden key to sustainable and adherable fat loss. You can't bunch together a handful of recipes and call it a solution to fat loss.

If you want a cookbook, fine. But if you want to understand the principles of fat loss for life, that's not going to help you very much. You might make a killer three-egg omelette, but you may also have Type II diabetes creeping around the corner.

Losing fat successfully isn't just about reducing the amount of body fat we have; it isn't just about storing less energy in adipose tissue; and it goes beyond improving health markers. When 'fitness people' are in debates they'll often hand pick certain improvements in health markers, which can sometimes be subjective. BMI, lipids, cholesterol or body-fat percentages are all commonly spoken about and debated in literature and now on social media, by experts and amateurs alike – delivering complex content and confusion to the consumer.

But fat loss, to me, goes way beyond that and much further than a six-pack.* It is:

- not worrying about what I order when eating out
- running with my top off because there's less wobble going on with each stride
- wearing something I wouldn't usually
- feeling good about myself
- starting a new sport
- waking up and being proud of my reflection
- spending more time naked
- lying in bed in the evening knowing I gave everything to every task I set myself for the day
- turning the lights on to have sex, not off

So my question to you: do you want to have less fat?

Good, but it's not *just* being less fat. You can tell yourself that, but it's bullshit. It's more than that. It's the fact that you wear black, the fact

---

* Everyone has rolls when they lean forward. I feel even people in good shape sit in the bath or on the toilet pinching their rolls of fat like they are alien – well, they're not; they're normal.

that when you stand up at work you pull your top down to cover your stomach. It's how not only your confidence is at an all-time low, but it's having a knock-on effect on other areas of your life – whether it's standing up in a meeting to express your opinions, going on holiday and worrying about the plane seat, or even what you order at dinner in front of your friends and a constant fear of being judged. It's about worrying about your health. We as human beings hugely underestimate the chances of bad things happening to our health or that of our loved ones.

This goes deeper than just weighing less. This goes further than having fewer cells with energy in them around our bodies.

Fat loss is about liberation, freedom, eradication of guilt, being more confident and not just looking better, but feeling better for every second of every fucking day. That's more than just having less fat, I can assure you.

Weight

Weight and fat are often used interchangeably. It's an issue I get pretty pissed off about, and I've moaned to clients about it over the years a lot.

James, I've lost inches, but I weigh the same as I did before.

Weight is your relationship to the ground with gravity, that's it.

The amount of fat you have is different and although over time there would be positive correlations between weight and fat loss, it's not to be taken as a metric to lose sleep about. Why? Because there are a lot of fluctuations in our weight which are not related to our fat mass.

To be crass, a long piss or a big shit could easily be enough weight in the bowel or bladder for you to step on the scales and pull your hair out. My personal record is about 0.6kg from a poo – I simply stand on the scale before, then again after. I've done the same when I really need a wee and I've racked up a similar weight. Imagine, if you will, you were to pee in a pint glass: if you fill it up, that's 0.56kg of water weight.

Ladies will fluctuate throughout their menstrual cycle, and you'll find out in the Female Fat Loss chapter (see p.261) that my female clients weigh Week 1 of their cycle vs Week 1 of their following cycle.

When people use the scale – or the 'sad step' – we have to be mindful of these **non-fat-related fluctuations**. If you're curious, fine, take a look. But there are a large number of you who, every time you decide to step on to the scale, then step off feeling demotivated, depressed and that your diet isn't working. And it's often because of these non-fat-related fluctuations. Sweat, hydration, muscle glycogen, time of day, bowel movements, fibre, salt intake and even how much you've had to speak (dehydration) – not to mention diuretics like coffee impacting on your net hydration – are all huge factors in weight. Considering 1lb (0.45kg) is enough for someone to be applauded or shamed at a slimming club, it's worth noting that although we should keep an eye on weight, it's a poor metric for short-term microman-aged 'success'. Month on month, it'd be pleasant to see linear progres-sions on net reduction of weight, but at some point that's going to stop and you're going to have to give it everything you have to lose half a pound.

So weigh yourself if you want to, because what gets measured gets improved, but please keep your emotions out of this. **Your self-worth cannot be quantified by your relationship to gravity.**

Some people will say to you that 'muscle weighs more than fat'. This isn't true. A kilogram of fat weighs the same as a kilogram of anything else, including muscle. Muscle occupies a smaller space than fat, though. So it's possible that in some people there will be huge changes to their shape and composition without their weight moving a huge amount over time. And that in itself is another factor to be wary of: the gravity we attach to our weight, pardon the pun.

At this point I should mention that without demotivating you, muscle growth occurs very slowly – much slower than you'd expect. So for men, play the long game; for women … any insinuation that you'll get bulky from lifting some weights is not only daft and unwarranted, it's statistically nearly impossible. Not only that, but muscle that could take years to build starts to degrade after only a few weeks of not training, so appreciate any that you do grow – after all, it will be short-lived if you don't maintain it.

Measuring body fat

If you want to know exactly how much fat you have on your body it's possible to find out – that is, if you're willing to be dissected. That's right: unless we can literally dissect you, there's no way of knowing exactly how much adipose tissue (body fat) you have at this moment in time. What we do have at our disposal are methods for getting good estimations of our fat mass.

The most common methodology for this is known as 'bioelectrical impedance'. Now, I'm sorry to break it to you, but this involves standing on plates placed onto scales and holding on to metal handles, so that electricity can pass through you to give off readings of all sorts, including fat-free mass, lean body mass and bone density, apparently.

Unfortunately, this is the least accurate of the mainstream methods to estimate how much fat you have; it's easily influenced by hydration statuses and, in my opinion, is a gimmick for gyms. Think of it this way: should your reading say you have more fat than you thought you had, you're going to think twice about cancelling that gym membership. On the flip side, should your body-fat percentage come out even lower than you expected – well, then you'd best keep your gym membership because it's paying off.

There are other means of measuring, such as a 'bodpod', which works by using 'air-displacement plethysmography', of course. Then we have DEXA, which stands for 'dual energy X-ray absorptiometry'. This was originally for testing bone density, and it's like a big X-ray that scans you lying down. Again, I often see these being used to determine how big someone is and to promote a macronutrient goal for that composition. Gimmicky again. (I never realized how long my femurs are until I had a DEXA, but although the experience was interesting, I don't think I'd ever really recommend one to a client, as I never got more than two sheets of A4 paper from it.)

Callipers are frequently used to quite literally pinch fat by creating skin folds. Although intrusive, they're actually measuring the distance between two parts of skin that are influenced by fat mass. Things like bloating, food in the gut and a few other variables can be reduced with this method. Eating a meal or drinking a protein shake would influence almost all measurements, but would not influence the callipers to a tangible amount as the fat between the skin folds wouldn't alter in that period of time.

Now, don't be fooled by plastic callipers that a PT at your local boot camp uses to pinch one area of skin and one area only. When calliper testing is done properly the locations on the body include arm, waist, subscapular (on the back) and on the legs in several places. The callipers themselves need to be calibrated and they're not cheap. Your boot-camp PT who got some plastic callipers off Amazon for £3 isn't going to give you an accurate reading, I can assure you.

When the measurements have been taken from the skin folds they're noted on a spreadsheet. The practitioner then needs to go back and do the measurements all over again in the same order, and should there be a sufficient discrepancy it will be done a third time. It's worth noting that you must go around the body before coming back to the initial measurement, due to skin elasticity changes.

Many variables, such as time of day and even time of week, must be maintained, and there are even variables between the people doing it, so you need the same person – in my experience it can take up to forty-five minutes for the test to be done properly. Even when using the same room to carry out the test, if the person is hotter or even slightly sweaty, it makes it harder to hold the skin to measure.

Although the percentage churned out from the reading may not be 100 per cent accurate, fluctuations in weight up and down usually are. So for instance, if you're 17 per cent, but the reading says 19 per cent, and you go on to lose 1 per cent in the coming weeks, although you'll read 18 per cent (but really be 16 per cent), at least you can roughly gauge the correct amount of fat that you have lost.

Now, someone has to pay for this, whether that's the trainer's free time or the participant's rate for the session. Plus, I can't help but feel that if you've just paid a large sum of money for a block of personal-training sessions and you don't see a change in the measurements, we could see some economy with the truth occurring. In truth, the reading says no change, the practitioner then proclaims, *'Well done. Albeit small, you lost … 1 per cent. That's great. Shall we go ahead with the next block of PT?'*

This is not to say there are no honest calliper readers out there. I'm just giving some context to one of the many issues I see in the realm of anthropometry (which is the nerd term for all of this). Another issue I see with the entire thing is the following hypothetical situation:

> John comes in to see me for a personal-training session; he confesses he's a lazy shite and needs to be more active and improve his diet. John knows he has 20kg to lose. I know he has 20kg to lose. He's a little apprehensive about the gym in general; he's worried about me judging him, others judging him and generally being outside of his comfort zone. I not only charge John a small fortune for the session, but before we even get going I am supposedly going to take him into a room, get him to undress down to his underwear and then pull away pinches of his fat before telling him he's got a lot of it.
>
> John will go home, his wife will ask, 'How was your first day?' He'll reply, 'Yeah, I got naked and had my fat pinched and recorded for forty-five minutes while I stood still.' He knows he has fat to lose – he's not an idiot.

This is not to say that's not how to do it – it's just not my approach. If it was up to me, I'd say let's leave callipers to those leaner populations who have much less noticeable fat reductions, who actually could need a reading.

We now know that scales can correctly track weight fluctuations, but are not necessarily representative of progress, and therefore not great for headspace and motivation. We have all kinds of rays, impedances and fat-pulling techniques, but what is the verdict from me?

Take a picture, mate. Since you got your smartphone a few years ago, you've taken pictures of your food every time you eat out, and each day you snap all kinds of photos you'd never have dreamed of taking before. Ever see someone take a picture of their meal with a disposable back in the day? Me neither.

My best advice for you to track your progress is to take photos. Let's imagine this is a scientific experiment, so let's try to keep any variables as similar as possible. These include time of day (I suggest first thing), location, lighting and hydration. These all play a role in this, so let's control these and any other factors that can influence the outcome as far as possible. I'm sorry to say it, but I've had lawyers, doctors and people in pretty important jobs telling me that they can't see a difference in their photos when there clearly is one. If you're not sure, you can always get another set of eyes on it.

You don't find good lighting; good lighting finds you.

Fitness 'Tracking' and NEATUP247

What gets measured gets improved.

This is not about food or drink. This is about movement. So if we revisit the bank-account analogy (see p.38), 'earning less' would be focused on changing the number of calories we consume. When we talk about 'spending more' we should not just be looking at training – this is a fundamental error that many people, including myself, have made over the years. I used to believe that the majority of my calories were burned while I was training in the gym, and that if I missed a session, the day was ruined and there wasn't even much point in trying to eat well.

What if I told you that maybe not even 10 per cent of the calories you burn today will be burned while training?

Would you believe me? Imagine a tower block with ten floors, where the entire building is going to represent the number of calories you expend in a day. Everyone burns a different amount of calories, depending on several factors, including weight, age and height and then how active they are.

Acronyms used to turn me off any subject. As someone who struggled in school, my brain switches off when I see them. BMR, TDEE, NEAT, TEF ... usually, my brain would make up the acronym NOPE (yes, I know it's not an acronym).

But I need you to learn this. Not for my benefit, *but yours*. If you understand this, then, quite simply, your quality of life when dieting

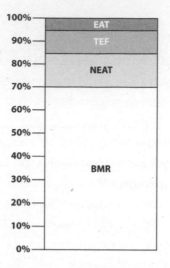

and training will improve. You will learn to move more and feel less guilty, and that's a recipe for a better life if ever I have heard one. Not just that, but again, getting your friends, family and loved ones to increase their NEAT (NEATUP247), as I'll explain in a second, can have profound impact on not just fat loss itself, but sustaining it too.

BMR

Seven of the ten floors are going to represent the number of calories you burn doing … nothing. Yeah, that's right. Known in the fitness world as BMR, which stands for basal metabolic rate, this is the number of calories you burn at rest. Seventy per cent of your calories burned today are burned without even moving.

Now, the last thing I want you to do is to suddenly think you don't need to get out of bed to get in shape or lose fat. I just want to make clear to you that missing a day at the gym is okay from time to time. I need to be real with you, and sometimes your kids, family or even friends will need you more than you need the gym.

Knowing that the majority of your calories burned each day occur outside the gym can liberate you to no longer feel guilt or a sense of failure when you opt to pass on it one day. Knowing what I'm about to teach you means that you could shave 10 per cent off your calories for that day and go to bed knowing you're still on track for success, rather than skipping the gym and heading down a spiral of a 'fuck it' mentality, eating everything in sight.

EAT

So just short of one floor of the ten-storey building (or 10 per cent of your daily calories) would represent calories burned through exercise, or exercise activity thermogenesis – EAT. This can, of course, differ between different types of training, effort and time spent, but typically, from what I've seen over the years on the gym floor, I'd say expending 10 per cent of your daily calories is the average. There are always the extremes of someone who has a photoshoot or a holiday spending 120 minutes on a cross trainer, burning 20 per cent of their daily calories and, on the flip side, Dave has just come in off the building site to do eight sets of bicep curls before hitting the pub, and may be lucky to expend 5 per cent of his daily calories – and that's before whatever he has at the pub. For every person over this amount, there will be someone coming in under it. Whether it be CrossFit, resistance training or a spin class, we consider all of these methods as 'EAT' – planned training; if it's in your agenda, it's in the EAT component (not the NEAT).

I've seen many clients over the years assume they're burning 500kcals in a session; truth be told it's more like 200kcals in the normal person who trains hard for an hour and burns 2,000kcals a day.

It's important to note the relative insignificance of EAT in the context of a day and, by extension, across a period of a week. The average 'fit' person trains only around four times a week, so it is crucial to focus on your NEAT every day (see below). I am not against training whatsoever, simply a pragmatist at heart.

TEF

Next up, we have (give or take) an entire floor allocated to the thermic effect of food – TEF. The TEF is the amount of energy expenditure above the basal metabolic rate due to the cost of processing food for use and storage. The thermic effect varies substantially for different food components. **For example, dietary fat is very easy to process and has very little thermic effect, while protein is harder to process and has a much larger thermic effect.**

This is another reason why 'high-protein' diets are advocated in periods of calorie restriction – its high thermic requirement during digestion. Around 30 per cent of the calories consumed in protein are lost/broken down purely in digesting it.

I've seen a meme that says, 'Studies show replacing carbs with protein but keeping calories the same results in fat loss – where is your calorie God now?' This shows a direct lack of knowledge surrounding the thermic effect of protein in the body and the positive effects it can have on fat loss.

NEAT

I'm about to change your life by explaining to you the NEAT component. Non-exercise activity thermogenesis – NEAT – accounts for calories burned outside of 'formal' exercise, such as standing, walking, climbing the stairs or even fidgeting.

Highly active people can expend up to three times more energy in a day than sedentary people. Although many people if asked would blame the obesity epidemic on sugar or carbs, I think it's important to note that the average person's NEAT has decreased substantially due to increases in motorized transport, sedentary jobs and labour-saving devices. Even an electric screwdriver saves your arm from burning calories when putting together your IKEA flatpack.

Ben Carpenter, a peer and good friend of mine, brought to light several studies on social media about NEAT and concluded:

When someone wants to lose weight, their initial instinct may be to go to the gym, which is great. However, maintaining an active lifestyle can burn a significantly higher number of calories than your average gym workout.

This has also helped demonstrate why some people gain less weight than others when overeating; they find themselves moving more when calories are increased whereas other people don't.

So, increasing your NEAT is free, simple to implement, has a low injury risk (compared to someone sedentary taking up running, perhaps) and can contribute a lot more to total calories burned than a gym workout performed a few times per week.

To be clear, I am not attempting to make a case against going to the gym, or implying that training is unnecessary. But I want to make you aware that movement outside of the gym needs just as much, if not more, consideration.

NEAT habits to have

Forming successful habits is crucial to hitting goals, and I'll expand on this throughout the book. Setting a step target or taking the stairs a certain number of times a day can have huge, influential impacts, not only on the amount of calories expended, but also as they positively begin to alter your attitudes and improve other areas of your life.

When I was personal training in Sydney we were two floors below the ground and the changing room was three floors below. I remember one day thinking to myself, How can I take myself seriously as a personal trainer if I take the elevator in the gym? From that day onwards, I never took the elevator and always took the stairs. It was a simple habit that I knew would have a profound impact on who I was each day.

To me, *not* committing to this habit could also have had a knock-on effect on other areas of my life: if I can't be arsed to take the stairs, can I be arsed to check my emails? From the second I implemented this I felt like more of an active person. Even if I was in the middle of a conversation with someone, I'd just say, 'Meet you at the top,' and, in most cases, I'd beat them up there, taking two stairs at a time.

From a fat-loss perspective, let's say I burned 5 calories on every stair run. I did that five to ten times a day, that's an average of 7.5 journeys. That's 37.5 calories a day, 262 a week and 1,000 a month. That's 3.4lb (1.5kg) of fat (hypothetically, each year) – and all because I decided to use my legs instead of standing still and checking Instagram amidst the awkward silence in a gym elevator.

Small habits like this make a profound difference to our identities. I make my bed every morning. And I make it well. I'm not even in the shower yet and I have a 100 per cent score streak on things I want to accomplish for the day. Should I leave the house with it unmade after I shower, I am only one out of two and have already ruined the chances of hitting a 100 per cent streak. The bonus is that if I hit a 100 per cent streak on all my daily habits, I get into a perfectly made bed every night.

Habits you can implement to increase your NEAT include:

- taking the stairs
- parking in the farthest space from the shops
- standing on public transport
- even when taking calls, you can put your headphones on and pace around the house tidying up or folding clothes

NEAT habits have substantial positive effects not only on fat loss, but on sustaining it too. Not only that, but it's so much easier to park in the empty part of the car park!

Over the years, I have honed a set of habits for myself. I can always trial new habits and ditch old ones, and **the actual habit is not as important as the outcome and impact of it**. Setting a reminder on my phone to supplement creatine has had a positive impact on my training performance, so the reminder remains. Setting myself a bedtime alarm to know to go to sleep has increased the quality of duration of my sleep. My current daily habits include:

- making my bed
- flossing in the shower and brushing my teeth
- packing my charger in my bag with my laptop
- leaving my bedroom how I'd like to find it
- emptying emails at 8 a.m./3 p.m.
- writing at least one marketing email
- posting at least one social-media post
- emptying all my WhatsApp conversations before 10 a.m.
- taking stairs where possible
- getting off my phone before 10.30 p.m.
- all devices on charge when I fall asleep

With all of these done, I can go into the next day able to do the same. It's not so much about each singular occurrence of the habit, but the compound interest accruing on their being repeated. Micro habits may not do anything for you today, but doing them every day, for years, can have huge and profound effects on your life.

Upskilling

I wanted to include upskilling within this section because it is a powerful habit.

A habit I have started recently is that whenever I've ordered food while I'm working on my laptop – whether it be breakfast or lunch – I think about the last tricky situation I got in while training in Brazilian jiu jitsu. I sit and think about where I struggled in a certain position sparring. I find a tutorial from a black belt where they explain that situation and the solution. I can't use my laptop as I eat, so I give myself ten minutes to watch, listen and learn. By the time I put my knife and fork together and push my plate to the side, I have learned something in what could otherwise be considered 'dead time'.

Sounds like a little bit of a loser thing to be watching YouTube instructionals when I should be enjoying my food, but it's a habit that's compounded over time to make me a better athlete. One day, it could be the exact concept I learned over my poached eggs, avo and sourdough that makes the difference between winning and losing a competition. Not only that, but think of the interest that would accrue over the years.

I have a saying, #alwaysbeawhitebelt. **If you think you know everything, you know nothing.** It's important to upskill, and although you may not be interested in how to get yourself out of a tricky jiu jitsu position, deciding to upskill your own expertise – for example, in a JSA module on how to barbell hip thrust or even an online tutorial about the anatomy of the hamstrings – might deliver a small amount of information at first, but the cumulative effect of upskilling over time could have a huge impact on your overall knowledge.

Tracking NEAT with fitness trackers

So where do 'fitness trackers' come into play? Nowadays, our smartphones, smartwatches or fitness trackers can tell us how many calories we're burning and how many steps we are doing each hour of each day. Personally, I don't advocate calorie tracking on these devices, as I feel there are too many influential factors for an accurate calorie burn to be recorded.

However, having something to make you aware of how much you're simply moving has a huge effect on fat loss in the long term. On days that we're incredibly active, we know about it; on days we're not, sometimes we don't even realize – and that is where activity trackers have their place.

Hypothetically: Sandra comes into the gym with her friend Sally and they both want to lose fat, so they begin a sensible resistance-training regime. They're the same height, weight, age and have the same job. Their calories, protein targets and training regimes are identical. They train together three times a week.

Sandra has a fitness tracker. Sally does not. Sandra notices a slight decline in her step count since adhering to the calories I've set her.*

Sandra, upon noticing the slight decline, opts to take the stairs at work, even when her co-workers are taking the elevator. She decides to take her dog for another walk each day, as she wants to keep her activity up to the level it was before meeting me.

Sally sticks to her calories, does her training and hits her protein target. Sally isn't really aware of NEAT and its impact on fat loss, so only really does what I've instructed her to.

Sandra will, for certain, see superior fat loss results to Sally because of this. NEAT is a crucial yet not widely spoken about element of daily expenditure and needs to be taken into account, not only by coaches, but by those being coached themselves.

During periods of calorie restriction, you may find yourself parking that little bit closer to the shops or less inclined to move so much. I certainly notice myself sitting at any given opportunity when I'm cutting calories. Being mindful of these habits and changes can help us prevent them from getting in the way of progress.

---

* One of the many adaptations to caloric restriction is subconsciously moving less; the further you diet someone, the less movement occurs. I've seen people who get very lean reduce the amount of gestures and fidgeting, and some even have noticed on camera that they blink less and slower. This isn't to do with our mindset or determination; it is usually out of our control, similar to an adaptation where we burn fewer calories, so therefore we produce less heat in a bid to conserve that energy, and many of my female clientele have noted 'feeling the cold more' during periods of caloric restriction – this makes total sense, as they have fewer resources to produce energy and keep themselves warm.

#NEATUP247

A special mention to Diren Kartal, one of my best friends and former JSA head coach, who has made famous the hashtag #NEATUP247 – his idea being for everyone to 'get their NEAT up 24/7'. This is a focus on people striving at every opportunity to increase their non-exercise expenditure, whether this is walking their kids to school, walking up escalators, taking the stairs or even the long route when going somewhere on foot. It's all about keeping your NEAT UP 24/7 – #NEATUP247.

I've already seen this change people's perceptions of their surroundings. Even at airports, where you have the moving walkways, I know people who now opt to walk to the side of them and shout '#neatup247' to their friends, like: 'C'mon, mate, don't miss out on an opportunity to get your neat up.'

I've been tagged on Instagram stories of people who say to their kids: 'What do we do here?' The kids run up the stairs shouting '#neatup247' to their parents. Non-exercise activity thermogenesis in a bid to promote subconscious energy expenditure is not the sexiest of subjects, but Diren* has not only got a substantial number of people moving, he has inspired them to encourage their family and friends too.

It's a positive movement and I hope one day we will have abolished the notion of being allowed to stand still on an escalator, if we are able to walk. There are thousands of people who would do anything possible for a set of working legs, so please don't take yours for granted: take the stairs, get your neat up and do it 24/7. After reading this chapter you'll have no excuse to neglect your NEAT.

* By the way, it's pronounced Deer-en, like Kieran with a D.

The tool belt – your 'secret' weapon

I often imagine a tool belt that we all have and wear each day, containing the tools we need to improve our overall lifestyle and aid us in reaching our goals. That might be, for example, increasing our NEAT one day to make up for a big hit of calories the day before, or some 'cardio' (which is EAT) because we're planning a big meal at the weekend and want to be able to eat that pizza.

I feel it's important to see these methods of burning calories, or reducing them in this way, at our disposal as our prerogative to use. Once we have the education to inform our decisions, we can choose and implement any tool whenever we like, or even opt not to use them at all. For example, having a step goal via a fitness tracker, albeit a non-essential addition to any person's routine, is a smart addition to someone's tool belt.

We can't wake up tomorrow and have much of an influence on the calories burned in our BMR, nor can we do much to affect the calorie content of our favourite foods, but what we can do is consciously increase both NEAT and EAT through attempting to move as much as we can when not doing planned exercise. Then, on the other hand, it's important we continue to make the most of our training and strive for a concept known as 'progressive overload'.

Progressive overload is where you seek and strive to make quantifiable improvements session on session, whether it's increases in weight or other metrics. I'll explain this in more detail later in the book (see p.257).

Other tools that we can use include food trackers such as MyFitnessPal, sleep-monitoring apps to quantify the duration of our sleep and even provide an estimate of its quality too. We can also work on conscious habits like parking further away from the shops or choosing to get off the bus or the train one or two stops early. None of these things *has* to be used; they're just there for when we need them. And it's always our prerogative to discontinue using them when we don't need them.

So always keep in mind your tool belt. A bit like a handyman who has at his disposal a tape measure, a hammer and a pen for when he needs one, you'll have your own tools, such as increasing your NEAT and tracking it on your Fitbit or iPhone, tracking your food on MyFitnessPal, doing an extra session in the gym, restricting calories for a short period of time to make up for a big social occasion …

You may find some tools more effective than others, but no two people losing fat are exactly the same. What you respond to best is for you to find out on what will be a journey of self-discovery. It sounds a bit hippyish, but there are a lot of things you don't know about yourself yet, and I want to help you find what you need, so I can come on that journey with you – not physically, but I'll be there in spirit, I am sure.

Habits – #gettingshitdone

Habits, in essence, form who we are. They make up our identity, but identities can change over time and it's important sometimes to remind ourselves of this:

> *'We are what we repeatedly do, therefore excellence is not an act, but a habit.'*
>
> Will Durant

No one is born with excellence. It's a skill, and skills are developed through repetition, often through creating a habit to repeat something. I have learned a lot on this topic from the author James Clear; he taught me that there are no bad or good habits – just habits that will contribute to our goals and those that won't.

Eating a doughnut is not a bad thing or a bad habit in itself; it's largely subjective. For someone who wants to lose fat, it isn't an ideal thing to be doing on the regular. However, for someone who is trying to improve their connection and relationship to food, that doughnut could be the biggest victory of their week or even month.

Up until the age of twenty-four, before becoming a PT, I hadn't actually accomplished much with my life at all. I was well travelled, had bad grades, no savings and I lived with my parents. Living with my parents was fantastic and I don't regret it at all, as it enabled me to throw myself full-on into my early years as a PT, with incredibly long days and lots of laundry. If I had to attribute any success since then to something, I would say it was down to creating solid habits.

A lot of what built my presence on social media was not so much what I posted about, but how I went about posting my content. Instead of worrying about how the post did, I just worried about posting every day. Instead of worrying about how engaging the article was, I just worried about writing it. I pencilled time in every day to write the articles and nothing would interfere with that habit. My following was below 2,000 for more than two years, but I kept my head down and just did my daily post and article. It was never about tomorrow's habit; only ever about today's actioned habit.

People ask me about my five- or ten-year plan, but honestly, I don't have one. I just worry about today. Tomorrow is influenced by today, so why even worry about it now? Today I have to write this book and I have to write a marketing email. If I don't do either of those, I will struggle to relax because it has now become such a strong ingrained habit to do them each day.

In my second year as a trainer, I came across a man named Paul Mort, who claimed that email marketing was the best way to make sales. I could not believe something as old-fashioned as email could be a medium for developing my business. Who the hell wants me to email them? I thought. Let alone every day. But Paul said daily vs weekly yields up to a 30 per cent better return on sales. I couldn't believe this until I signed up to his paid plan – because he emailed me every fucking day until I cracked!

I now run one of the world's largest email lists in the fitness industry – one of the most profitable too. I email several-hundred-thousand people each day with something entertaining that has nothing to do with fitness, then pitch for business at the end. In LA, earlier this year, I got stung $500 for a laundry bill and my first reaction was: 'This will make a good marketing email.' Not only profitable, but therapeutic – I'd never have known that, having originally thought it was the most boring medium for marketing.

I started my list with one email to one subscriber. I didn't worry about growing the list, I didn't worry about sales; all I worried about was setting and ingraining the habit. **Focusing on the habit is crucial – it's not about the instant gratification that comes with effort.** The reason most personal trainers fail to build an online presence is because they create a habit and expect an instant return on the investment of effort, and if they don't see one, then they discontinue the habit. They do not let the habit work over time to yield a substantial return.

THE ICE CUBE METAPHOR

In his book *Atomic Habits* (see References, p.285) James Clear speaks about an ice cube in a room. It sits there and nothing happens. You raise the temperature by one degree, still nothing happens. Again, another degree, nothing happens; another degree and absolutely nothing has happened. But all it takes is one degree above freezing for it to begin to melt. We should keep this analogy in mind in life and not expect our ice cubes to melt immediately after changing the temperature by a degree or two. You need to focus on it degree by degree – maintaining steady habits to achieve change.

Since I decided to write my daily emails, all I have done is focus on writing them each day. I just got on with it and learned along the way. Now, three years later, I have proof that committing to something every single day has yielded a positive response and a growth of my community and business.

Olympic lifting is all about repetition; there are no short cuts to getting a good snatch or clean and jerk. You must input hundreds of hours and thousands of repetitions, and rest assured that behind great success is a trail of mistakes, lessons learned and small improvements.

Do you know how long it took me to make my first sale via email? Ten months. Ten months of writing an email every day.

At the cost of 5.8 days of solid email writing (thirty minutes per day) for ten months, I made £20 on my first sale. That works out at 14p per hour for my efforts as an email marketer. Not something that many would aspire to on paper. Hundreds of days with nothing in return – just notching the temperature for the ice cube up a degree, so to speak. I posted online for two to three years before I ever got an online client too.

People can't believe how many emails I send, and they ask me what the trick is to grow an email list. I tell them: thirty minutes of your time every day, *for years*.

You cannot email someone too often; you can only be too boring.

It's worth noting this too: people who accomplish great things in life and those who accomplish little to nothing *often have the same goal*. I've been working online as a personal trainer for several years, and I'm sure there are a lot of others who aspire to do it and never will. The difference does not sit within my ability to speak publicly or create engaging content; it sits within my daily habits.

So an aspiring athlete and a gold-medal Olympian have the same goal. These will relate to sleep, nutrition, training and life in general. One of my Brazilian jiu jitsu training partners got a gold medal in the Olympics. He told me that every time it pissed it down with rain, he'd go outside and sprint. I asked him, 'Why?' He told me that every person he'd ever come up against in the Olympics would be inside, out of the rain, which made it the perfect opportunity to get one up on them while they remained dry. That sounds like the habit of a gold medallist.

If we take this approach into a training scenario, this could be about setting a habit of training in a certain area of the gym, ensuring you're using a particular piece of equipment and making it habitual to step outside your comfort zone, increasing that discomfort and gym-based anxiety no more than one degree at a time. Before you know it, you could hit the metaphorical melting point for all your insecurities and worries in the gym, using the squat rack unassisted for the first time. And I'll bet you could do all of that without having to worry about getting your socks wet like my Olympian friend.

My favourite quote from *Atomic Habits* is this:

'You should be far more concerned with your current trajectory than with your current results.'

James Clear, *Atomic Habits*

And this is where I need you to take note. **Where you are is not important; where you are going is.** You may not have the body you want, you may not have your diet in the place you want it. But are you getting better at taking action to make those changes? If so, great. Are you making progress? If so, great. And if you're not making progress, are you making adjustments so that you soon will be? That's what is important here.

You could well finish this book and not have made physical changes to the point that someone will notice them just yet. But that is okay. Rather than worry about your current situation, just worry about your current trajectory. You'd be amazed what you can accomplish. **Successful habits make successful people.**

Think about my trajectory with my email marketing list. It was always improving, although I had nothing tangible to show for it. Yet the thirty minutes a day I put aside for this way of communicating with my clients could just be one of the greatest habits I have ever implemented. One email a day, in time, will pay my parents' mortgage off, so they have more of their retirement money to live with until the end of their days.

Writing emails has become very therapeutic, almost like keeping a daily diary. However, do you know what made it easiest for me? I have fallen in love with the process of writing an email each day, so rather than it being a burden, a task or a chore, it's quite simply a habit I enjoy doing.

My advice to you: **find your successful habits, implement them daily and then fall in love with executing them**. You'll stumble across great success just from that alone.

Habits in practice: flexible dieting and IIFYM

It's a good idea to expand on these terms commonly mentioned in the fitness industry. You may have heard of flexible dieting from fitness people or you may have heard of the 'if it fits your macros' movement (IIFYM). I'll clarify the differences. I have touched on macronutrients briefly before. But essentially, the idea of tracking 'macros' is to set yourself goals to hit each day to get what is optimal* from your diet, which is commonly known as a 'macro split'.

Fun fact: adding up your macros equals your calories. With protein at 4 calories a gram, to consume 20g of protein would equate to 80 calories.

IIFYM

I alluded earlier on to the fact that athletes and fitness people have often been misled about what is a 'good diet' and what is a 'bad diet' for them. For years, I've seen confusion over what is an optimal amount to eat (and even when to eat), and this is the case even with people in very good shape playing at elite levels of sport. I have found over the years that the best athletes tend to do so well through their attitude and determination within their field, but I've been very surprised to see what some fantastic athletes actually eat on a daily basis. Some have such a poor understanding of nutrition, it's actually crazy. By the end of this book, you'll be better clued up than most Premier League football players.

The origin of IIFYM comes from what I can only assume were conversations between coaches and their clientele. 'Coach, can I eat pasta?' And the response: 'Sure, **if it fits your macros**.' 'Coach can I eat some bread today?' The response again: '**Sure, IIFYM.**' A bit like, 'C'mon, mate. I set your macros – if it fits, go for it.'

Now, this IIFYM mentality did great things and evolved into the term 'flexible dieting'. I'm sure the Pareto principle of 80/20 was thrown around a lot too in Internet discussions – 80 per cent good

---

* Optimal is subjective here. Personally, I think that someone hitting their macronutrient target vs just a calorie target is essential to optimize their return from tracking in the first place.

food, 20 per cent junk – but, unfortunately, IIFYM over the years has been interpreted as: 'Eat shit but make it fit your macros and you'll be fine.'

This isn't what anyone ever intended with this concept. Now, of course, you're always going to find people who abuse any system and don't do very well – in the same way that I'd very easily abuse the 'intuitive eating' lifestyle by interpreting the guidelines so that I can eat whatever I like: 'Oh, mate, I had three burgers today, but if I drink six scoops of whey protein, it will fit my macros.'

There are many more complex components beyond macronutrients that are essential to looking and feeling good and living a healthy life: food quality, unprocessed 'single-ingredient' foods, vegetables, fruit, fibre, variety – these all contribute to our health and make up the essential vitamins that we need. Another component is food volume. I always ask my clients to expand their food choices by selecting lower calorie foods that could increase the amount on their plates. This would typically include, for example, more vegetables, rice, fruits and leaner meats and protein.

However, what I have found is that following macronutrient goals gives people the initial momentum for improvements to their diet. I've found that even just setting a protein goal alone has seen a spontaneous improvement in the quality of the diets of my clients over the years. I'd also back the fact that even just being mindful of caloric intake, whether divided into macronutrients or not, would have a massive impact on the amount of food you eat.

When I give a regular person, who could be very new to dieting or even tracking their food, a mid-tier protein target, suddenly some form of planning has to occur, and it's very rare for someone – even if they are new to eating in either of the aforementioned manners (IIFYM or flexible dieting) – to sit down with their family with just a chicken breast on their plate. More care goes into the intake of the food, and that is compounded over time.

A lot of this game is about being mindful of our food consumption. All too often we eat out of boredom, or because something catches our eye, or a smell gets us interested as we walk past a bakery. For thousands of years food was scarce, and although the food industry has a target on its back, of course they'd be silly not to make calorie-dense foods, hedonic by nature, very appealing to the eye and the taste buds (after all, they say the first taste of your food is in how it looks).

And I don't think we can criticize or abuse the food industry for doing this. Everything is about marketing – whether it's putting sprinkles on a doughnut or making yourself look good to 'market' yourself when asking a stranger if they 'come here often?' But being conscious of your goals and aware of the calorie content of certain foods, even when something appeals to you, will strengthen the argument in your head to say what's most difficult in the world of fat loss: 'No thanks, I'm good.'

If I were to use my James Smith Academy calculator online I could get a macronutrient split back that may look like this:

'Thank you for using the James Smith Hypothetical calculator, your macronutrient goals are: **190g protein, 44g fat, 200g carbs.**'

So to translate the macronutrients into calorie totals:

190g x 4kcals per gram + 44g x 9kcals per gram + 200g x 4kcals per gram = 1,956 calories

That'd be my 'macro' goal.

NOT A DIET BOOK

Flexible dieting

Flexible dieting and IIFYM can be used interchangeably, but I personally have an alternative take on how to do it.

My version of flexible dieting is a slightly different approach to dividing your macronutrients up and how you prioritize what to structure first. What I get my clients to do is assess and then implement everything in order of importance. Of course, for someone looking to lose fat, the bottom of the pyramid is calories. It shouldn't matter how much of each macronutrient you're consuming if you're not hitting your calorie target.

Protein is the second key player here. You'll find out a lot more about protein in this book, but it plays a big role in muscle growth and fat loss. You'll have a very tough time at either end of the spectrum, whether your goal is muscle growth or fat loss, should you not get enough protein.

Carbohydrates and dietary fats are both energy sources with their own respective benefits, but when it comes to looking to lose fat, you can select what suits you based on personal preference.

I find IIFYM a very rigid and strict structure compared to my preferential 'flexible' approach. Again, this probably depends on the person. If you are someone who loves numbers and works in tax and accounting, you might like the idea of having numbers to aim for each day. Someone like myself, who'd rather get caught up over two numbers than three, might prefer the more flexible approach. To give you an idea of what I mean, let's use the same macro goal as before:

190g protein; 44g fat; 200g carbs

Ideal scenario

▸ **Calories met closely** 1,956 = *c.* 2,000 each day or even *c.* 14,000 weekly.

▸ **Protein met closely** 190g = as close to 190g as possible each day.

▸ **Carbs and fats** = remaining calories after protein to be split according to personal preference, but ideally, do not eat a very low-fat diet (typically, I'd never recommend going lower than 20 per cent of total calories from fat).

Not-so-ideal day

▸ **Calories met, slightly overshot** = if overshot, implement reduction over following days.

▸ **Protein under hit** = next day, try to do better, maybe add a protein shake.

▸ **Carbs and fats** = next day, try to be more calculated with which energy macronutrient you prioritize – for instance, if you have an evening training session and the next day you're training early, it would make more sense to consume more carbohydrates to help you fuel the following day's session.

Bad day

Like a majority vote we don't need every day to be a winner, just the majority. Keep in mind that people who are in good shape for a living rarely get long streaks of success without a bad day; they often just call it a 'cheat day' to mask the fact they've had a bad day. We can't expect our diet to be good all the time – it never is. It's just about getting more good days than bad days.

Train wreck of a day

Make a mental note or an approximation of calories consumed or don't even track at all if personal circumstances are bad; remember that saying – 'one hot day doesn't make a summer'.

SUBOPTIMAL   OPTIMAL

Your position can be anywhere within the many shades of success, and everything becomes more of a spectrum of suboptimal to optimal rather than black or white, good or bad, success or failure.

So you will sit somewhere on this spectrum with both your diet and your training every day. All we want to do is move towards the optimized end of the spectrum whenever possible. The truth is, you never really need to be fully optimal. To live that life you'd have no alcohol, go to sleep at 8 p.m. every night and probably never have children. If we all aimed for a perfectly optimal life, it would be pretty boring. The reason I prefer a more flexible approach is so that some days it's okay to give your diet less attention and focus, and that is fine – it's a part of being human.

All I want from you is to implement some processes each day, those habits and whatever you do to bring you in line with being as optimal **as possible**. I don't expect you to hit your protein every day, but try on as many days **as possible**. I don't expect every training session to be spectacular, but keep it as intense **as possible**.

Truth is, things get in the way of an optimal world. An argument with your partner, feeling under the weather, rain on the way to work when you're late already. This is all about getting the best possible scenario each day and not beating yourself up if you have a bad one; it's not wasted, it's just suboptimal.

The main objective is to get more days optimal then suboptimal. It might sound oversimplified, in which case I'm glad, because it's true, and it's attainable.

Essentials for the Good Life

In this section of the book we're going to get into the nitty gritty of things **I need you to learn**. They may require some rereading, but I would not have included them if they weren't essential for you to 'live your best life'.

Hopefully, you've got all the 'tools' you need on your tool belt at your disposal (see p.70) now, but there are also some elements that are integral to life, and which you need to ensure are in order. So hold on, buckle up and read carefully – these next bits will change your life for the better.

Vitamin D

We get Vitamin D from being in the sunlight – hence it is also known as the 'sunshine vitamin'. It's bloody excellent for us for many reasons, and I would never leave 'getting sufficient sunlight' out of general advice when talking about optimal health and wellbeing.

Vitamin D is technically a 'fat-soluble vitamin'.* It's used by the body for bone development and increases our ability to absorb calcium, magnesium and phosphate. A healthy circulating level of Vitamin D is greater than 30ng/mL†.

---

* Fat-soluble means that it is absorbed with fats and can be stored in fatty tissue.

† This will help people determine how many 'IUs' they'll need to take when supplementing Vitamin D – an 'IU' being an international unit. Ng/ml stands for nanolitres per millilitre.

It's estimated that a billion people worldwide have a Vitamin D deficiency. This is mainly attributed to lifestyle, where people are not spending enough time outdoors, and this can sometimes be influenced by environmental factors such as air pollution and even work shift patterns.

Inadequate amounts of Vitamin D are not only a public-health issue, but a worldwide epidemic. We're starting to see the development of rickets (a skeletal disorder) in some children, which is very concerning. There was even talk of getting Vitamin D put into the UK water supply because so many people are deficient.

You can supplement Vitamin D to increase your intake because it is rarely obtained from any foods, unlike most other essential vitamins. Weakness, fatigue, aches and poor bone health are symptoms of being deficient in Vitamin D. Not getting enough plays a part in developing osteoporosis, which is the degeneration of bone health.

The association between depressive disorders and Vitamin D deficiency from a lack of sun exposure is well established and was first noted 2,000 years ago. Awareness of Vitamin D has grown exponentially over the last fifteen years. New mechanisms and diseases associated with deficiency of sunlight include cancer, cardiovascular disease, diabetes and premature mortality.

Sunlight exposure and Vitamin D supplementation have proven to have a similar effect to some antidepressants. Now, I am not saying, 'Oh, if you're depressed, just get more sun,' but it's certainly a factor to consider when looking at potential causes for depressive thoughts or symptoms.

An interesting study found that weekly doses of 50,000IU of Vitamin D (D2) in women with Type II diabetes who had significant depressive symptoms and low Vitamin D levels **resulted in an improvement in**

depression, anxiety and mental-health outcomes. (See References, p.285). I'll be covering diabetes in much more detail later in the book – see p.111.

I certainly feel a lot better in environments where I am exposed to sunlight, and I get at least fifteen minutes in the sun each and every day. My physique, mental health and even my ability to learn have come on leaps and bounds since following the sun from hemisphere to hemisphere. I know it's not an option for everyone, so if you can get sun, get it, and if you can't, I highly recommend looking into supplementing Vitamin D.

Again, I'm not insinuating that if you're fat, depressed or both, you should just sit in the sun and you'll be fine. What I am saying is that it should not be overlooked as a very important part of your lifestyle and overall health. If you are not sure of your levels of Vitamin D, you can either take a test or supplement for a few months to see what differences you notice.

I'll be recommending Vitamin D in several sections of this book. I have no discount code or commission code – just look into a way of supplementing a few months' worth. And I'd love to hear how it plays out for you!

Sleep

When looking back at hugely important elements of my life I overlooked, I'd say sleep is at the top of the list. I can't emphasize enough how, since learning about its impact on health, state of mind, performance and even sticking to a diet, my life has changed. I suppose I never gave any thought to the reason why we sleep or the repercussions of not getting enough. Now I focus on my sleep as much as on putting fuel in a car – without it I quite simply cannot perform or concentrate as long with daily tasks at work and training.

So many people are looking to supplements and 'superfoods', training regimes or quick fixes to enhance their current situation, but little do they realize that there's an almost magical solution out there that can boost recovery, performance, cognitive function, sex drive and help them stick to a calorie deficit. And even better, it costs nothing – **it's quite simply getting enough sleep**.

I want you to imagine two massive pyramids of important things in your life: one is essential for general wellbeing, and the other for achieving your diet and fitness goals. I don't believe that the latter can be achieved effectively without first implementing and understanding the former.

Whether your goal is to perform better, gain more muscle or be slimmer, sleep plays a huge part and should be one of the first areas to audit.*

---

* By 'audit', I mean you should take a moment to step back and reflect on your habits and see where improvements could be made. You could audit your diet or food log and look for improvements of food swaps, for example.

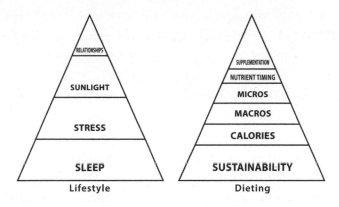

When auditing sleep you want to look at duration for a start. There are some apps on smartphones, and Fitbits can also gauge the quality of the sleep you get. Audit your sleep log for the last seven nights. On how many of those nights did you get seven to nine hours?

Although sleep is free, there is certainly a place for investing in it with the right mattress, pillows and your sleep set-up in general, which might include fitting some better blinds for your room and a fan to keep you cool during the summer. I say to my clients, 'Yes, it costs the same as your holiday that you went on for a week, but ultimately, you'll spend years and potentially a decade going to sleep in that set-up each night – and that's a better return on investment than a week away in Turkey, all-inclusive!'

Personally, I love to have a soft mattress, and I need more pillows than you could shake a stick at. In recent years, I have, funnily enough, become accustomed to sleeping with a pregnancy pillow. Sounds odd, but it cost me the same as two gin and tonics and it's revolution-ized my sleep quality – I often find myself waking up in the exact same position I went to sleep in. Something so simple from Amazon has had such a positive impact on my daily life, and I'm sure that any investment you make in your sleep set-up will be returned. I also have a fan in London and Sydney at the ready for a warm night; it's much easier to fall asleep when you're a little bit too cold than a little bit too hot. Cost per use – you're laughing at the end of the day.

It is essential that you strive to get seven to nine hours' sleep every night. Yes, seven to nine! Not six, not five. **Seven to nine!**

The average person in the UK wakes up at 7.35 a.m. – this means that to get nine hours you'd need to go to bed and be asleep by 10.35 p.m. I need you to trial this for me as soon as you can – tonight, if possible. Even if it means putting this book down right now. I'll be here for you tomorrow when you've had enough sleep.

Getting adequate sleep will benefit your fat loss, your muscle growth and even your libido.

Fat loss – quite simply we're more likely to overeat when we're sleep-deprived, and we make poorer food choices.

Muscle growth – testosterone is a key player in muscle growth in males and females and is drastically affected by our sleep duration and quality.

Libido – both the factors of body composition and testosterone will also have a profound influence on our libido and sex drive. So all the more reason to improve your sleep habits, which affect these two factors.

Lack of sleep and overeating

In a study, binge eating was reported by 244 (6.4 per cent) women and was positively associated with not getting enough sleep, sleeping poorly, problems falling asleep, feeling sleepy during work or free time and disturbed sleep. These same sleep variables, as well as napping and being a night person, were also significantly associated with obesity. (See References, p.285.)

Lack of sleep and testosterone

'Daytime testosterone levels were decreased by 10 per cent to 15 per cent in this small sample of young healthy men who underwent one week of sleep restriction to five hours per night, a condition experienced by at least **15 per cent** of the US working population. By comparison, normal ageing is associated with a decrease of testosterone levels by **1 per cent to 2 per cent per year**.' (See References, p.285.)

To reiterate, a 10 to 15 per cent decrease in just *one week*, with those rates of decline correlated with a decrease we see of roughly 1–2 per cent a year with age. By reducing your sleep to five hours a night for one week alone can add ten years to your age in relation to your libido.

Looking across a meta-analysis of research, we can conclude that testosterone can have anti-depressive benefits. I think it's very important that we start to make a correlation between sleep deprivation and low testosterone (although it's not the only cause) and see the importance of this hormone not just for performance and function, but for self-esteem and mental health.

Testosterone is sometimes categorized as the 'male sex hormone'; however, it is produced by both men and women – men more so – and fluctuations in either sex can have a big impact on libido and performance. It can also have positive effects on mood and muscle mass. Many men can feel emasculated through reductions in testosterone. Losing your libido can have a huge knock-on effect on mood, daily life and mental health.

Testosterone replacement therapy (TRT) is growing in popularity in the USA. Anyone who has below what is considered 'normal' amounts of testosterone can qualify for TRT. However, nowadays it's common practice for people to quite literally trick their doctors by manipulating test results. The reason people do this can stem from wanting to maintain their physique as they age, and can include all sorts of people, from amateur athletes to corporate gym-lovers.

The European Male Aging Study (EMAS), a population-based survey performed on more than 3,400 men recruited from eight European centres, has clearly shown that sexual symptoms – **decreased frequency of sexual thoughts, decreased morning erections, and erectile dysfunction – are the most sensitive and specific symptoms in identifying male patients with low testosterone**.

Hence, **illness-related, obesity-related or age-related hypogonadism** (characterized by a failure of the testis to produce and release adequate concentrations of its 'products' i.e. sperm and sex steroids – testosterone) **are not recognized as true pathological conditions needing a pharmacological intervention**. The recently published Guidelines of the Australian Endocrine Society fully endorsed the FDA's position, **suggesting that removing the underlying metabolic conditions, such as losing weight, must be the optimal therapeutic strategy** for treating obesity-associated hypogonadism, and that testosterone replacement therapy is not justified in such conditions. (See References, p.285.)

To conclude, sleep is far more important than just how you feel when you wake up; it can – and does – have huge implications for the production of testosterone and the associated repercussions (mood, libido, morning erections and erectile dysfunction). If you're not waking up with a boner, it's time to get on top of your health.

Sleep rhythm and hormones

Sleep is a biological process that is essential for basic functioning, but also for optimal health. **Sleep plays a critical role in brain function and systemic physiology, appetite regulation and the functioning of immune, hormonal and cardiovascular systems:**

What physiological issues can we face when not well-slept?

- ► **Physiology** – what substrates* are used in a deficit, fat vs muscle mass
- ► **Appetite** – the ability to adhere to a calorie deficit
- ► **Immune** – increased chances of getting ill when undersleeping
- ► **Hormonal** – testosterone and other vital hormones that are affected by sleep
- ► **Cardiovascular** – the impacts on sleep and heart health

Circadian rhythm: sleep hormones

So now I'm going to talk about something that all of us have – even our pets. It's a circadian rhythm – our body's cycle that allows us to fall asleep when we're tired, and prompts us to wake up in the morning. It's something that a lot of you, before reading this chapter, will have taken for granted and never realized why it is that jet lag, for example, messes us up so bad.

There are two hormones you need to know about: **cortisol and melatonin**.

---

* Substrates here refer to muscle and fat tissue; both can be broken down to be used as energy should it be needed.

Cortisol

Cortisol has a bad rep within the fitness industry (and outside of it), but I'm telling you now it's important, and although branded as the 'stress' hormone, it's actually essential for daily life and homeostasis (the condition of optimal functioning, or the 'dynamic state of equilibrium' within the body). Basically, for balancing things out for optimal health.

Cortisol is one of the hormones that we produce to help us get out of bed; this is known as the 'cortisol awakening response'. Unfortunately, this is why, often, when you wake up hungover, or try to have a lie-in at the weekend, you can't simply fall back to sleep when you want to. The rhythm plays to your advantage to get you out of bed and into work each day, and you can't simply shut it off as easily as you can your alarm. Incidentally, you'll note that on days you go to bed on time and don't set an alarm, you wake up at roughly the same time. This is due to your sleep rhythm. We usually only oversleep an alarm if we've had a late night or have messed up our sleep rhythm through international travel.

Throughout the day, cortisol maintains blood glucose (aka blood-sugar levels). In addition to its paramount role in normal daily function,

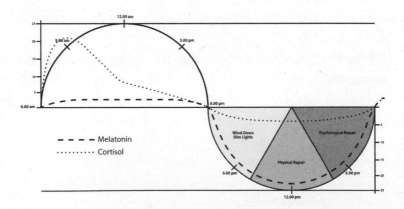

it is a key player in the stress response. In the presence of a physical or psychological threat, cortisol levels surge to provide the energy (and substrates) necessary to cope with stress-provoking stimuli or to escape from danger – otherwise known as the 'fight-or-flight' response.

Unfortunately, in the modern world it is quite common for this hormone to do its job more than it should. Social media, worrying about emails, things popping off in the group chat on WhatsApp – even when you come home to watch a gripping TV series. These all play into your hormonal response from cortisol, which can make it difficult to fall asleep. I talk about Brazilian jiu jitsu later on in the book, but it's worth noting that a lot of people struggle to fall asleep after sparring because of the adrenal/cortisol response making it harder to get enough good-quality sleep.

So to conclude, cortisol is good. Without it, we couldn't try to outrun a bear or simply wake up in the morning. 'Managing' your cortisol is about as stupid as managing your insulin (as long as you're not Type I diabetic, that is).

Melatonin (mela-toe-nin)
Melatonin is the hormone that helps us fall asleep.

Remember the first time you were told that caffeine would improve sports performance of any kind and it became your go-to every time you needed to perform well? Melatonin is the complete opposite and is your go-to when trying to sleep. Supplementing it can also help you stabilize your sleep rhythm when travelling.

When flying long-haul, you have probably heard that going one way feels a lot worse than the other. This is because getting jet lagged one way means we have to stay awake longer, but we can use things like sunlight, caffeine and keeping active to stay awake and 'push through'. Unfortunately, there are not so many external aids to help us fall asleep without having to look to sedation through things like alcohol – and even then, there's no guarantee you won't wake up halfway through that sleep due to your body and circadian rhythm thinking it's just a nap.

Human beings have been on the planet for hundreds of thousands of years, but it's only within the last century or so that we've been able to cross through several time zones in a day. Unfortunately, we cannot expect our sleep cycle to adapt to these advances in modern-day travel.

Disturbed circadian rhythms are associated with sleep disorders and impaired health.

So what does melatonin do?

Melatonin regulates circadian rhythms such as the sleep–wake rhythm, neuroendocrine rhythms. Ingestion of melatonin induces fatigue, sleepiness and a diminution of sleep latency.

When circadian rhythms are restored, behaviour, mood, development, intellectual function, health and sometimes seizure control can improve. (See References, p.285.)

I began supplementing melatonin and found it hugely reduced my 'recovery' time when flying between Sydney and London. It's worth noting that in Australia especially, the shelves in pharmacies are full of 'homeopathic' remedies, which don't always contain what you would get from a prescribed supplement.

If you suffer from the effects of jet lag, go to your doctor and they will prescribe you the good stuff.

Each person is going to react slightly differently to sleep deprivation, and the majority of people who are sleep-deprived don't even know it. So someone who is constantly tired and fatigued may not feel the effects of jet lag too much due to that being their norm. However, someone who is used to waking up well-rested and going to sleep on time (like myself) will struggle with the altered cycle of sleep when abroad.

As soon as I get on the plane I think about how I need to adjust my circadian rhythm as soon as possible through melatonin supplementation. Even if this is part placebo, I am a believer that if a placebo works, it works. I look at the 'world clock' function on my iPhone, and if it's time to go to sleep where I'm going, I take a few melatonin and try to get the cycle on track ASAP.

Melatonin supplementation is slow releasing and allows us to sleep for up to nine hours, or even longer. Having insufficient melatonin in circulation makes it very difficult to sleep for that long.

The reason I have included melatonin in this book is that it's another tool on your belt, counteracting the effects of long-haul travel, whether for business or pleasure. It's another way of taking back control, contributing to optimal lifestyle habits.

> *'If you don't sleep the very first night after learning, you lose the chance to consolidate those memories, even if you get lots of "catch-up" sleep thereafter. In terms of memory, then, sleep is not like the bank. You cannot accumulate a debt and hope to pay it off at a later point in time. Sleep for memory consolidation is an all-or-nothing event.'*
>
> Matthew Walker, *Why We Sleep*

Our brains work with two systems: a cognitive system and an automated one. What I want you to think about is when you first learned to drive and you had to think of every movement: clutch, lift, accelerator, press. Before long, everything moved into system 2, whereby it was automated, feet moving without cognitive effort.

In the sport of Brazilian jiu jitsu I prioritize my sleep, especially when I increase the amount of training. Not only is it imperative for energy and for my body to repair, but also to be able to remember what I have learned. Only since learning more about sleep can I look back and see the benefits of getting a good sleep routine alongside my training.

Sleep disruption

Disruption of sleep is something of a concern too. Sometimes just going to bed at a certain time is not enough to ensure adequate quality of sleep.

A 2014 survey conducted by the National Sleep Foundation reported that 35 per cent of American adults rated their sleep quality as 'poor' or 'only fair'. Trouble falling asleep at least one night per week was reported by 45 per cent of respondents. In addition, 53 per cent of respondents had trouble staying asleep on at least one night of the previous week, while 17 per cent had been told by a physician that they have a sleep disorder, which, for the majority (68 per cent), was sleep apnoea. (See References, p.285.)

I think it's a good idea here for me to categorize disruption and deprivation together in a similar context because the negative outcomes remain the same. It's important to improve our understanding of what can have a detrimental effect on our sleep, not just for ourselves, but for those around us. If I catch any of my friends ordering a coffee at a certain time in the afternoon, I'll remind them: 'Hey, mate, it's 5 p.m. you realize? Bit late to have a coffee and you may struggle to sleep.' They may then opt to have something else to perk them up, like a cold diet soda, which has a fraction of the caffeine content.

I am not a sleep zealot. I just used to be the person who drank evening coffees to keep me going when training people at the gym and never quite understood why I couldn't fall asleep.

Lifestyle disruptions

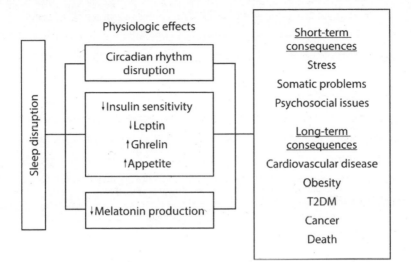

Caffeine

I'm not going to say that caffeine is by any means 'bad'. Athletes perceive weights to be lighter under the influence of caffeine, and without it I would have skipped a lot more training sessions in the past few years. There's also a high chance I wouldn't have been able to write this book without an abundance of coffee.

My main concerns with caffeine are centred around timing; should it disrupt your sleep cycle if you consume it too late in the day and hinder your ability to fall asleep, that's an issue. The other element I object to is when someone uses caffeine to mask genuine fatigue or 'overtraining' (see p.188). Sometimes an early night and a good night's sleep will do more for someone's fitness journey than a forced training session fuelled by a huge amount of caffeine, which could all too easily lead to another night's disrupted sleep and feeling more tired still the following day, and so on.

Caffeine affects people differently. My parents have a cup of coffee before bed and I'm confused about why they do it to this day. It is thought that there might be up to 33 per cent of people who do not respond to caffeine ingestion. (See References, p.285.) However, this might be an over-extrapolation of the current data due to the fact that I'm sure more people will be forthcoming about not responding to caffeine in comparison to those who do feel its effects. It's just something to keep in mind. I'm sure if I left a pot of Vegemite out on the side, more of my friends who disliked it would comment than those who liked it.

Alcohol
For years, I thought that booze helped you sleep – a nightcap, as my dad would call it. Unfortunately, this means the period you spend in bed is more sedation than sleep and usually hinders the body's natural sleep cycles. This isn't to say you should never drink; just be warned of the effect. Nowadays, I avoid the odd 'one-off beer' because I am conscious of the detrimental effect it could have on my sleep – that's me, though: a typical not-drinking or all-in kind of person.

Drug abuse
As narcotics such as MDMA and cocaine become more widespread, people are often staying awake for much longer periods than their circadian rhythm would like, and the health implications include not just the effects of the drugs themselves, but the associated sleep deprivation too.

Shift work

Now, I honestly would love to label this part of the book 'GET A NEW JOB', but unfortunately, shift work is essential to society. Doctors, nurses, service-station attendees, flight attendants, pilots, police, ambulance crews, firefighters and so many more are crucial, and we need people to be working shifts.

From what I have learned about the importance of sleep, it's clear that shift work will only hinder the balance of someone's circadian rhythm. This is not to say that their life of training and dieting is wasted, but we have to be mindful that the effects of shift work are 'suboptimal'. At the end of the day, it's important to keep in mind that if you're not quite getting the energy to hit every gym session at every intensity you'd like, ultimately your profession is more important than how you look on the beach. Even fitness models can't all afford to support a family with their six-pack alone, so sometimes we have to realize we can't have both.

As we can't realistically eradicate shift work, I think that more needs to be done for those who do it. Ideally, a shorter working week or something to compensate for the fact that they're constantly going to be tired and never fully on a proper sleep cycle – even giving them a four-day week and a longer weekend to recover. I don't think throwing more money at the problem is a good enough solution to this big issue. We need a better understanding of the negative impact of shift work. Nurses, doctors, etc. will be more likely to make professional mistakes if they are sleep-deprived and, ideally, we should shorten their shifts and the number of days they work. Shift workers, in my opinion, should focus on creating the best routine surrounding their sleep; if anyone has the choice to do shift work they should always opt for more sensible hours, but in cases where it's not a choice they need to ensure the sleep they do get is of good quality and duration.

Jet lag

This is the term commonly used for circadian changes caused by long-distance travel. As I mentioned before, we can travel over several time zones a lot faster today than ever before. Our circadian rhythms have not adapted and evolved as fast as our technological advancements, so we experience extreme bouts of 'catch up', whereby our biological clock must fall in with the rest of us.

This must be taken into consideration, especially when seeking caloric restriction (dieting). Being jet lagged makes everything hard: waking up, going to sleep, adhering to a deficit and, most of all, resisting food cravings. When I travel long-haul and am suffering from jet lag, I can't stop eating everything in sight.

If you have to travel a lot for work, or you change time zones frequently, the bottom line is that it will influence the outcome of any dietary interventions you implement and could potentially lead to health issues later on in life that are associated with lack of sleep. Alzheimer's is being connected more and more with sleep deprivation, and I think we're going to see more research in this area in years to come.

It's important to reduce the impact of the negatives associated with jet lag by being mindful of the circadian changes and ensuring that you try to get some form of rhythm back as soon as possible, whether by using melatonin (see p.97), setting bed and wake-up times that suit the new time zone or pushing back to your boss for more time off when you are suffering with jet lag.

Light

Melatonin helps to regulate the circadian rhythm as discussed earlier (see p.97). Production of melatonin in the brain is under the influence of the hypothalamus, which receives information from the retina about the daily pattern of light and darkness.

The reason we have curtains and are advised to stop using phones or screens at night is that bright lights influence the production of melatonin.*

Screen time needs to be managed when considering sleep, especially in children. More modern models of smartphones have features such as 'night mode' to prevent the problems associated with bright light and melatonin production, but we also have to take into account the effects of being cognitively dialled into a device when we should be winding down.

I know many of you might be thinking, **James you haven't had kids! What is sleep?** Is that Spanish? With children, my best advice is to take into account what you have just read about light and melatonin, timing of caffeine intake and sleep patterns, and implement what you can, where you can for a better night's sleep for you and your kids. Prioritizing your child's sleep could have a positive impact on your own too.

Sleep apnoea

Obstructive sleep apnoea is a potentially serious sleep disorder in which breathing repeatedly stops and starts. It is an under-recognized and underdiagnosed medical condition, with a load of negative consequences for health. Symptoms usually include daytime sleepiness, loud snoring and restless sleep. Undetected sleep apnoea can lead to hypertension, heart disease, depression and even death for someone who would be at a much-heightened risk of falling asleep behind the wheel (see References, p.286).

Several forms of treatment exist for treating obstructive sleep

---

* A test called Dim Light Melatonin Onset (DLMO) is used to measure whether someone's melatonin output is healthy. (See References, p.285.)

apnoea, including continuous positive airway pressure (CPAP*), oral appliances resembling mouth guards, which help with breathing during sleep, and surgical procedures. However, more conservative approaches such as weight loss, discontinuation of drinking alcohol and smoking are also strongly encouraged.

Sleep apnoea can be linked to weight gain. As you can imagine, there is a vicious circle of someone who gains weight through some sort of life event – whether it be a change of job or a mix-up in routine. Their sleep cycle is then disrupted by the onset of sleep apnoea, which, in turn, causes them to feel sleep-deprived and more likely to consume more calories the following day, causing the sleep apnoea to get worse. If you suspect sleep apnoea, it's important you see a doctor; if you're diagnosed with 'excessive sleepiness' you must inform the DVLA, who may prevent you from driving.

Sleep and fat loss

So why is all of this important to you and your fitness 'journey'? When looking at insufficient sleep and reducing the amount of fat someone has, the statistics are, quite frankly, worrying:

'Sleep curtailment decreased the fraction of weight lost as fat by 55 per cent and increased the loss of fat-free body mass by 60 per cent. This was accompanied by (…) adaptation to caloric restriction, increased hunger, and a shift in relative substrate utilization towards oxidation of less fat.' (See References, p.286.)

In *Why We Sleep*, Matthew Walker draws attention to how people in sedentary jobs, such as truck drivers, struggle to expend enough calories due to the nature of their work – they're often sleep-deprived,

---

* CPAP is a type of ventilator that keeps the airways continuously open, and which some people require to get proper sleep.

driving at times to avoid traffic and, because of their food choices when stopping on the road, they are more likely to consume far more calories than they require for the day. This puts them in pole position to develop obesity and, therefore, sleep apnoea. And this means that when they do finish their shifts, they're not going to get good-enough quality sleep, putting them at a much-heightened risk of falling asleep behind the wheel the following day.

> *'When you're drunk your reactions are slowed, meaning you brake late in an accident, but when you're asleep you don't brake at all.'*
>
> Matthew Walker, *Why We Sleep*

So although many people have a pop at office work or the traditional 'nine-to-five', just think that you're in a strong position to obtain good quality sleep. Your job or commute may give you a headache sometimes, but it's not something to take for granted. You have a consistent work cycle, which means implementing a consistent sleep cycle is not going to disrupt your work.

If you ever moan about making it to work for 9 a.m., just remember most personal trainers have their first client at 5.30 or 6 a.m. We'd almost consider a 9 a.m. start the afternoon!

For some reason, humans have recently, whether intentionally or not, started to sleep-deprive themselves with no real knowledge of the repercussions to health and state of mind. I use several means of ensuring I get at least seven to nine hours of sleep whenever possible, and have listed them for you below:

▶ **Setting an alarm to go to bed** Although this sounds a bit weird, I often set an alarm to remind me to go to bed. It's usually about an hour before I plan to be asleep; this means if I am flossing, brushing or getting stuff out the washing machine, I can start doing it way before I need to be asleep. You may think you're really organized, but I promise this will make a difference if you implement it yourself. I know you may have children or a partner who's not fully on board, but the return on investment here is huge and it's something you can do for yourself right now.

▶ **Audiobooks and podcasts** There are timers on both of these if you scroll down on your smartphone. I often set mine to eight or fifteen minutes. Not only do I drift off to sleep easily, I do it learning, and I often wake up remembering some of the last things I listened to. Podcasts are a lot easier, as usually people are having more formal conversations. I even purchased a small Bose speaker to take with me whenever I am travelling. When I travel with Diren (founder of NEATUP247, see p.69) we share a room and we often face conflict when I set the timer for fifteen minutes and he wants thirty minutes instead – funny thing is, he rarely reaches the ten-minute mark before dozing off.

▶ **Caffeine** I have a cut-off of around 3 p.m., sometimes 4 p.m. for this, after which I then choose to wake myself up using another method that I'd consider 'good for the soul': when I'm in Sydney, that's a dip in the sea; in the UK, it may be a random shower,* partly with cold water. (I can't quite get on board

---

* Over the years, whenever I've struggled for inspiration, a concept or content ideas, I have had a random shower. Even topics for the book have come about while having random showers, and I keep my phone near me for the Notes setting to transcribe my ponderings in the shower. Give it a go if you need creativity.

with the 'cold-shower movement'. I flick it cold for about seven seconds, then squeal and go back to the original and much warmer preferred temperature before getting back to work.) It's worth noting that decaf coffee isn't zero caffeine; it often contains up to 30 per cent of the caffeine content of regular coffee.

▸ **Magnesium and lavender spray** Now, although I don't think there's much solid evidence backing the claims, I know anecdotally that some people sleep well using this. It's something for you to try. And remember, if a placebo works, it still works. I used to use magnesium to help me sleep, but recently I have not had any problems sleeping.

▸ **Sleep apps** Remember: what gets measured gets improved. Maybe setting yourself some goals could improve sleep habits and, therefore, sleep patterns.

Understanding Diabetes Mellitus – For Everyone

I first became interested in diabetes when I was only three months into personal training and I took on my first Type I client, whose name was Sam. (It's quite rare for someone to develop Type I at an older age – she was about thirty.) Diabetes is not part of the syllabus when qualifying as a PT, so whatever I write here comes from what I have learned over the years since, and Phil Graham, who is a Type I educator, peer and friend in the fitness scene, has always answered any questions I have, so I'm very grateful for his input. Here, I'm going to share what I think is a useful amount of knowledge on the subject and break it down in the best way I can. Whenever I break something down, I literally convey it in a way that I have communicated with myself in order to understand it. I nearly left this section out of the book – I know it's not light reading, but in the next few years (or maybe already), someone close to you may have some form of diabetes and you can have a positive impact on their life by understanding it.

I do not wish to underestimate the seriousness of diabetes in any way by attempting to oversimplify it in this chapter. I am just trying to communicate the understanding I feel you may need at this stage.

So what is diabetes?

Diabetes is a group of metabolic diseases characterized by hypergly-caemia,* resulting from defects in insulin secretion, insulin action or both. The long-term hyperglycaemia of diabetes is associated with long-term damage, dysfunction and failure of different organs, especially the eyes, kidneys, nerves, heart and blood vessels.

Diabetes comes in several forms – four, to my knowledge, although I only really want to discuss two of them here: Type I and Type II.

► Type I – results from the pancreas failing to produce enough insulin.
► Type II – is a condition of defective insulin signalling.
► Gestastional – a condition where women without previously diagnosed diabetes exhibit high blood glucose (blood-sugar) levels during pregnancy, especially in the third trimester. Please consult a doctor for more information on this.

It's estimated that right now over 400 million people are living with some form of diabetes, and most of us just don't know enough about it. I spoke to a man on the Tube recently and he told me he was Type I diabetic. I bombarded him with questions (I am fascinated by the complexity of it). I asked him what living with it was like, and he told me he often got judged by people around him for having it. This is because people jumped to the conclusion it was lifestyle or poor deci-sions that had led to his condition. However, this isn't always true, and I

---

* Hyper means a lot of (as in, hyper-active); glycaemia means 'the presence of glucose in the blood': hyperglycaemia = too much glucose in the blood.

feel it's largely unfair and unhelpful to tar everyone with the same brush when it comes to diabetes.

It actually pissed me off that people are so quick to assume what type of diabetes he had, so I want to dedicate this part of the book to all those who have to live with diabetes and the unwarranted judgement that can come with it.

Type I

Typically known as the 'insulin dependent' form of diabetes. This is an autoimmune disease where the body attacks itself. Some of the other most common autoimmune diseases I've come across with clients include Crohn's and rheumatoid arthritis.

Type I diabetes develops as the body attacks the cells in the pancreas responsible for producing insulin. If insulin can't control blood-sugar levels and do its job in bringing glucose out of the blood, the glucose levels in the blood begin to rise, causing hyperglycaemia.

When someone with Type I continues to eat, especially carbohydrates, their blood-sugar levels are hiked high at the same time that cells in the body are not getting the fuel they need, or the glucose out of the bloodstream. The body will often start producing ketones. (If you remember, earlier in the book I spoke about ketosis occurring when glucose availability gets very low – see p.27.) Although there is a lot of glucose in the blood during hyperglycaemia, it's not available, so the body begins producing ketones. Although ketosis isn't immediately harmful, when excessive levels of ketones and glucose circulate the bloodstream for long periods, people can suffer the life-threatening state of ketoacidosis.

Type I can be managed with administration of insulin and using blood-glucose monitors to check when blood sugar gets too high or too low. Over time, Type I diabetics can learn when they need to administer and how much during certain feedings.

The cause of Type I diabetes is still not known fully, and I am sure you can see my frustration as to why many people don't have a choice when it comes to Type I diabetes.

Type II

This is the most common type of diabetes. The fundamental issues seen with Type II are insulin resistance and reduced insulin production. Being pre-diabetic is a term often used to describe patients who are at risk of developing Type II if they do not change their lifestyle or habits.

Family history, poor diet, being obese and sedentary put you at highest risk of developing Type II diabetes. I believe it was called 'adult-onset diabetes', but unfortunately now we're seeing it in younger populations, and even teenagers are developing Type II diabetes.

The reason for the rise in obesity is complex, and I'd be misrepresenting it if I said it was just because we 'eat too much and don't move enough', but our environment is growing evermore sedentary. It's deemed an effort by most to even meet their Deliveroo driver at the front door; at least not so long ago we had to walk to the chip shop to buy our fish and chips! And Uber means that we walk less, while some physical jobs are being replaced by technology, especially in the industrial sector worldwide.

The key to reversing pre-diabetes or improving symptoms and effects of Type II must be to exercise as often as possible and to reduce body fat by implementing what you learn throughout this book. Increasing insulin sensitivity is the goal, and I'll talk about it more below.

INSULIN RESISTANCE

Insulin resistance is primarily an acquired condition that is related to having too much body fat, although there are other causes linked to genetics and conditions like polycystic ovary syndrome (PCOS), which I'll explain more about in the female fat loss section of the book (see p.261).

What I often tell my clients is: *'When there is an inability for your body to properly respond to insulin, you're insulin resistant.'* The most common causes are obesity (which is having more fat than you need). Other factors can be age, lack of exercise or a sedentary lifestyle. Training a muscle will increase insulin sensitivity at the muscle site; this is because even with insulin resistance there will be glucose (often stored as glycogen*) being 'used' as fuel at the muscle, meaning more demand for more fuel to re-enter the muscle to replenish it.

Keto and Diabetes

It's quite easy to draw a conclusion that following a keto diet means lower levels of insulin and therefore a solution, right? Although ketogenic diets are becoming more popular and some people are experiencing tremendous amounts of weight loss (with removal of many hedonic foods), I could therefore get behind a Type II using the protocol; however, the very low amounts of carbohydrates (often 20–50g per day) they could run

---

* Glycogen, as we learned earlier, is carbohydrate stored in muscles. I like to think of a muscle as a sponge, and when you train it you squeeze it. Then it has the ability to soak up whatever it can (carbohydrates). Should you not squeeze a sponge, no liquid will leave it, so it cannot take in any more.

the risk of a Type I experiencing a 'hypo', which would lead to issues with sustaining long term.

Exercise not only means burning more calories, which is great, but it also increases insulin sensitivity to muscle tissue. Imagine on one end of the spectrum you have insulin resistance; what you want is to increase insulin sensitivity.

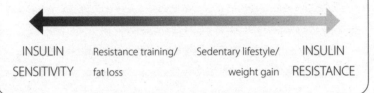

| INSULIN SENSITIVITY | Resistance training/ fat loss | Sedentary lifestyle/ weight gain | INSULIN RESISTANCE |

You're not obese because you're insulin resistant; you're insulin resistant because you're obese.

Unfortunately, the daily habits that are formed over the years to make someone pre-Type II diabetic or even Type II cannot simply be undone by medical intervention. Giving them a handful of pills isn't going to change the habits that have been ingrained every day for years and sometimes decades.

When setting goals for weight loss it's hugely important to make them small. For instance, like I've said before, you don't have 10kg to lose – you need to lose 1kg; that's all your focus needs to be on – 1kg at a time and nothing more than that. When you've lost that 1kg, it's time to set your sights on the next.

Treatment of Diabetes Mellitus

Treatment for diabetes aims to keep blood glucose levels as close to normal as possible to reduce the risk of developing complications. Treatment will vary depending on the type of diabetes. Lifestyle modifications in conjunction with medications like insulin are often needed. (See References, p.286.)

> *'Effective management of diabetes is a team effort between the person with diabetes and respected and suitably experienced health professionals.'*
>
> Phil Graham, *The Diabetic Muscle and Fitness Guide*

For anyone who has more complex queries, especially those associated with Type I diabetes, I would advise following Phil Graham, who is a fitness business coach and has also helped me with this section of the book:

@philgraham01

Please always seek medical advice if you have, or suspect you have, any type of diabetes.

Laws of the Universe

I want not only to set the foundations that you require for the smoothest journey in changing parts of your identity, body and mindset, but also to arm you with a new way of thinking, new perspectives and to save you from the tricks your mind can occasionally play on you.

I want to make you reassess your thinking about physical change, mental growth and how you approach new information. From here, you can wipe the slate clean and bring clarity to your thought processes and, ultimately, decision making, for good.

To explain the potential impact of all this, I'll tell you about the time one of my mentors got me to implement changes in the way I dealt with my clients. He briefly explained to me Pareto's 80/20 rule and, in essence, I identified that 80 per cent of my headaches, frustrations and annoyances came from 20 per cent of my clients.

Just by applying that simple law to my business a few years ago, I managed to erase 100 per cent of my headaches for only a 20 per cent reduction in my salary. People are intrinsically biased towards not wanting a reduction in their income – not only from a practical point of view of having less money, but also because we've been taught to associate this with failure. But it's time to rethink this. Never having to deal with the clients who pay late, turn up late and don't appreciate your time for a 20 per cent reduction in pay and 20 per cent more time to work on my business – that was a bargain, and just one of the many laws I have applied to my life which have, in turn, made both my work and personal life much more enjoyable.

The Confirmation Bias expanded

The confirmation bias is a term coined by English psychologist Peter Wason and refers to the tendency to search for, interpret, favour and recall information in a way that confirms your pre-existing beliefs or hypotheses (see p.42).

In simple terms, **we buy into the things that back our own beliefs and disregard those that go against them**. I'm now much more aware of this, as should we all be, within all areas of our lives. It's so easy to remember whatever supports that which we're already thinking and disregard anything that challenges or doesn't fit in with it. I often say that 'I'm Switzerland' in debates or conversations about certain diets or topics of discussion: I don't like my bias to affect the outcome, and neither do experts, scientists and researchers when working on studies.

It's important that all bias is left behind and doesn't interfere with data. Some research, for example, is conducted using 'blind studies', where the participants don't know if they are taking a real drug, a supplement or just a placebo, so that their bias cannot affect the outcome, nor are they susceptible to suggestion.

For instance, I could give two of my friends a fizzy drink. One has caffeine in it, one does not. If I told my friends they both had caffeine, I could observe their performance in a workout to see the difference. However, there would be a slight bias, as I know which one really had caffeine.

A 'double-blind study' is one in which neither the participants nor the experimenters know who is receiving a particular treatment, drug or supplement. Double-blind studies are particularly useful for preventing bias. So in this instance I'd give both friends the fizzy drinks without even knowing myself who had which. This would eliminate any bias from me too.

> *'People are forever saying "you can find a study to support any belief". The truth is, no you can't.'*
>
> Martin MacDonald, nutritionist

Visit any gym and often you'll see a personal trainer dishing out advice to their client based on what worked for them. If the PT does low-carb, all their clients will do low-carb. If the PT does fasted cardio, all their clients will do fasted cardio. These people have usually fed their own existing bias, whereby they accrue data to support their belief and disregard anything that challenges it. So from now on I'm asking *you* to challenge it. If you put the effort in to find what works for your own long-term goals, rather than following the latest fad, you'll be empowered and gratified – and you'll be able to help others spot any bullshit that's being peddled too.

The sunk cost fallacy

The sunk cost fallacy is another trick of the brain, which I realized I'd succumbed to a lot in my life after learning about it in *Thinking, Fast and Slow* by Daniel Kahneman. It's also briefly covered in the Rolf Dobelli book *The Art of Thinking Clearly* (see References, p.286).

So what is the sunk cost fallacy?

The Misconception: you make rational decisions based on the future value of objects, investments and experiences.

The Truth: your decisions are tainted by the emotional investments you accumulate, and the more you invest in something the harder it becomes to abandon it.

What this means is that we often irrationally make decisions based on the wrong factors, one of the most prevalent being how long or how much we've already invested in it. The more money, time, effort or even sacrifice given to a task, person or investment, the harder it will be, ultimately, to walk away from it.

The sunk cost fallacy is the reason you have the gym membership you don't use, why you find it hard to leave the slimming club you have been with for years and why it's hard to discontinue the direct debit you have with a diet app.

Through this entire book I'd like you to challenge yourself on certain areas of your life, from your PT, your diet and your training regime, right up to your relationships – I mean the ones closest to you, perhaps your partner or spouse.

I'm going to ask you straight: how is the relationship you are currently in? Is it serving you still, daily? Are you married – how is that? Are you still having regular sex? How is it?

You're probably wondering why this PT is butting into your personal life, but this is very important. Have you ever thought or considered that the quality of your relationship has a direct influence on the amount of calories you are consuming each day and how much exercise you are doing – or not doing – each day?

Straight away, I'll usually hear a defensive, 'Yeah, we're fine, we're great.' But over the years, I've challenged my clientele and asked them:

'If your relationship was like it is now when you first met, would you have stayed with that person?'

Now, I'm not just being nosy. I'm here to delve a little deeper than simply 'eat less, move more' and find out what's going on subconsciously, contributing to why you picked this book up in the first place. Just as the taxman may audit you for financial discrepancies, you can see me as the curious PT, seeking the potential underlying issues, small or large, that are standing in the way of you and your progress.

Through several years and thousands of hours of training and coaching, relationships have cropped up as an area to be explored further. People fall victim to the sunk cost fallacy in their own homes, and the worst bit is that they often don't even know it.

Living under the same roof with your boyfriend or girlfriend in a sexless existence of bickering and arguing makes them more of a flatmate than a soulmate.

I can't help but think that too many people who are sharing a mortgage with someone think they're in a successful relationship because they're on the property ladder – and that's just not right. Remember the frog in hot water analogy (see p.32)? Well, that's most relationships I have come across: slowly heating up and no one even realizes how hot it's getting because the temperature rises so slowly.

When I have to tell someone that they need to move on and break up with the flatmate or 'partner', they'll say something like: 'But we've been together for four and a half years.' Then I have to tell them the harsh truth and reality of the situation – that they've succumbed to the sunk cost fallacy.

The amount of time you have spent with a person should not impact on the decision of whether or not you should be with them now.

The harsh reality is that you need to act on how things are **now**, and whether or not that relationship is serving you. Not them, but you. We can sometimes find ourselves worrying too much about others – how they will be, how they'll cope – and I'm afraid that when you're on a journey of bettering your own life you need to put yourself first. Sometimes your partner/flatmate/mortgage contributor is creating drag on your progress, like poor aerodynamics, ultimately slowing you down and making it harder to move forward. This is about YOU, not those around you, not yet – we can help them later, but work on yourself first.

I'm no relationship guru, but I'm a firm believer that we need to be selfish in life, to look after ourselves first, to perform daily actions that make no one but ourselves happy. Don't get me wrong – being selfless can make us happy and improve our moods too, and, ironically, we can do kind things for others just to make ourselves feel better and that's great. But the key thing here is that I think both parties in a relationship need to be equally selfish with maintaining their own happiness, health and standards – and then bring those two positive entities together to share a happy life.

I see people coming home from jobs they don't love into relationships they're not passionate about, but they are not pragmatic enough to just call it a day, to end it, to endure the heartache and change. Humans hate change by nature, but sometimes it needs to be done. Think about this … Is it any wonder that people who don't get anything from their job or relationship turn to food? It could quite literally be the thing that brings them the most pleasure in the day. It's fucked to say that, but it's true. Sexless relationships aren't healthy because often one of the parties will be thinking, I'm not attractive or good enough. In some cases, this can cause one of the partners to change, but all too often it leads to them doing nothing – to them, the sexless existence of being together becomes the norm.

Another unspoken element of imbalance in a relationship is within what I call 'spouse sabotage'. For analogy's sake, let's say in a relationship where both parties earn the same amount, if one gets a pay rise, it could easily disgruntle the other. Coming home to celebrate the household net earnings going up should logically be a positive discussion. However, it can leave the person without the pay rise feeling inadequate, that maybe they're not doing as well as the other person.

Similarly, when someone in a relationship wants to make changes, it's often not always supported by the partner, despite what they might say. The progress of the partner who starts to lose fat and comes home to celebrate their weight loss or measurement decrease can all too easily leave the other party feeling inadequate, like they should be making changes as well. In some cases, this can motivate them to follow suit, but more often than not they – subconsciously or not – end up trying to sabotage the efforts of the dieter to bring things back to normal, to how they were before.

The psychology required for someone to decide to make change, to sort out their exercise and dieting regime, is unique, and it doesn't always fit in with the agenda or priorities of the person they're in a relationship with. Both partners will have different values and habits; we can't expect that just because one of us wants to do something the other will too. Not to mention how it must feel for the person left behind. So what is easier for that person to do: to catch up or sabotage the partner's efforts to bring them back to the norm, how they were before, without change?

In relation to fitness, a common theme that hugely disrupts the headspace of a woman in particular is the notion of being 'too muscular'. When it comes to strength training, women can worry about gaining too much muscle and perhaps not looking feminine enough for societal norms. The hormonal profile for a female makes muscle growth depressingly slow and difficult, which, in itself, means this notion is hugely irrational. It's a bit like if you were to open a savings account with a small amount of money and then worry about becoming a millionaire by accident. I have come across the scenario many times in which a partner has said, 'You're getting too muscular, too muscly. You have arms like a man.' I could pick a thousand things that are wrong with this, but the main one is that never in my life have I seen a woman's arms that are 'too muscular' – and I know girls who have been to the CrossFit games and can pull themselves up a rope without using their legs. I would never in a million years dream of saying they're too muscular.

It doesn't take long to lose fat compared to building muscle. However, the repercussions of losing fat can make someone look more muscular very quickly, and it can often annoy the person who is making no progress – the partner, for instance. So their response can sound like this: 'You're training too much.' Or, 'You've become obsessed with fitness, it's not healthy.' Or, 'You've got too muscular; it's like going for a walk with Arnie.'

These types of comments can come from loved ones and family members, but also friends from a wider social circle. And, whether intentionally or not, they can cause the process (or attempted habit change) to be disrupted.

I'm sick to death of women having to worry about the false notion of getting too muscular just because some insecure males can't handle the fact that their girlfriends are getting their shit together while they're at home doing nothing for themselves. It winds me up so much whenever I come across any insinuation of a woman being too muscular. Lifting weights makes women strong. Being strong often plays over into a woman's world outside the gym, which can be liberating. For someone out there to potentially stop training due to the words of a jealous spouse should not be stood for.

To all women reading this: if your partner has ever said or says to you that you're too muscular, I'd start looking for a new one. You're better than that and you deserve better too. There is someone out there who will support every aspiration you have in your fitness journey, so never settle for less than that – it's quite literally not good for your health.

Insecure men are poisonous for the growth of an aspirational woman.

Friendly fire, friendly sabotage

You've probably experienced the following scenario with some of your friends before: my best friends and I have a term we call 'secret dieting', and it's when we catch one of the others out for beginning a fat-loss diet without telling us about it. When we catch wind of it we actually become annoyed, outraged that one of our best friends, right in front of us, has begun a diet without acknowledgement or support from us.

We'll order food, then their meal will turn up and it'll be a salad. Outrage. 'A SALAD? Are you secret dieting?!' The interaction that follows will mimic Denzel Washington in the film *Training Day*, where he feels like everyone has turned on him and hung him out to dry. I'll just wait until I get home and send ten McDonald's McFlurrys over to their home address. That'll cost me just over £10, and if I get a 20 per cent hit rate, that'll add 300–400 calories onto their daily total, rendering their salad utterly useless. Watch out for secret dieters, they are the worst types of friends.

Now, a point I want to make clear is that with my friends it's banter and often harmless, as we're all best friends. However, sabotage within relationships can become toxic, and when looking at its repercussions, I think we could even consider it abuse – physical and mental – which is not to be taken lightly. My friends and I are all of healthy dispositions and we would never intentionally cause distress to each other, but it can happen a lot, and with malice.

It's very rare to find a couple who don't share similar daily habits, and most couples who become obese often do so together. Eating habits, similar diets and usually a joint sedentary lifestyle can lead to very fast weight gain, which becomes a taboo subject between the couple in question. 'Shall we just get a takeaway tonight?' all too easily becomes a joint justification.

Imagine for a second you're speeding down a long, narrow lane. You're doing 70mph, although you know the limit is 60. Now, in a similar scenario, there's another car in front doing 70; suddenly, it becomes more acceptable to keep up with that car. If they're doing it, surely you can too? People tend to match the speeds of the surrounding vehicles because not only do they feel like they fit in, but **the more people do something together, the more acceptable it is**. You don't have to look further than a gathering with friends to see how overeating occurs and is considered absolutely fine as long as others are doing it.

Often, beginning a diet or proclaiming a change in dietary habits can bring about a situation where you'll hear something like, 'Sure honey. Sounds great.' But really the wheels are just about to start turn-ing to bring you back to the shared baseline. 'Oh, you look fine, have an ice cream with me, it's only one, anyway.' And there are so many other cues, habits and shopping lists that will sabotage your efforts. Without your partner's 100 per cent full support you will revert back to old habits.

Maybe they don't want to diet, they don't want to train, they don't want to change. I'm afraid that the love of your life (so far) could be one of the biggest hindrances to your ability to sustainably make change in your life. The person sitting next to you or opposite you as you read or listen to this could be the very one who needs to either adapt and support you in what you want to accomplish or face the repercussions and become a part of your past, alongside your old lifestyle, exercise and eating habits.

To summarize: take a good look at your existing relationship before you delve into the following chapters. I think the author Mark Manson says it best when he says:

'If it's not a fuck yes, it's a no.'

If you thought it was easier to stick to a new diet on the first day of the year, imagine what it'll feel like when you quit the job you hate, dump the partner you are no longer in love with and become a happier, more confident and active version of yourself. It's time to cut your losses on anything that's going to slow you down. Be ruthless, be selfish – because ultimately, as I said before, this is about you.

Powerful shit, right? It's like *Game of Thrones* the James Smith way. No one is safe – apart from your dog. We like dogs.

The Power of Numbers

What a boring topic, I hear you think. Listen, I know it sounds bad, and I'm not the type of guy to wank over complex algebra either, but honestly, we're going to cover off numbers, and when you see 'The James Smith Game of Numbers' in the same way I do, everything will be much simpler.

When I finished university with no degree and quite literally nothing to show for the horrendously large fees for 'education', I was living with my friends and my old man, Geoffrey Smith, essentially cut me off. Each month, he'd very generously sent me £100 for beer, sausage rolls or the odd emergency taxi. But one day, I looked and the money wasn't in my bank account.

I called my old man and he said to me, 'Son, you're no longer at university. You're an adult now – you can go get a job if you need some money.' He had a bloody fair point, but I remained in denial about the entire thing. I waited a week, maybe two, played a lot of games of *Call of Duty* on my Xbox.*

I vividly remember telling my dad there was 'no work available' wherever I looked for it. He said to me something I didn't think I'd have to hear, not in a million years – something that was going to rock me harder than losing a game of *Call of Duty*. He said to me, 'Son, go sign on the dole. I've paid enough bloody tax for nearly fifty

---

* If I could have converted my skills on *Call of Duty: Modern Warfare* to the real world I could have made a good living, in hindsight.

years, so you may as well see some of it back. That's what it is there for.'

I wasn't happy about this suggestion because it made me consider how hard (or not) I'd been trying to get a job, and I didn't want to lean on the State unless I really had to. However, rent needed to be paid and sausage rolls needed to be bought. Oh, yeah, and beer too. So, I went to the Gloucester Jobcentre, located near where I lived at the time, and experienced one of the most uncomfortable situations I have ever been in.

I was asked all kinds of questions and I found very quickly that if I wrote three lies on an A4 piece of paper in my finest writing, I could get the State to pay all my bills and I could return to a life of *Call of Duty* domination. However, I opted to use one of the touch-screen machines and I printed a ticket and took the first job going. Within six weeks, after training and driving my dad's Rover 75 Estate to Worcester every day, I was finally a 'Sales Representative' for npower.

What was I selling? Gas and electric. Who was I selling it to? People who already had gas and electric. How was I selling it? Knocking on fucking doors all day, every day.

I took my £12,000 annual salary, and with a spring in my step, I hit the doors for what would end up being bloody months of door knocking to make a living. Waking up each day and knocking away. Two sales a day kept my manager happy. I was fortunate enough not to be in a team with someone micromanaging each knock, and instead I was able to do my hours as I pleased. Some days I'd be home by 2 p.m., others I'd be soaked through with rain and going home with nothing in commission, telling my boss I'd had a tough day.

I'm not sure many postcodes in the UK could beat GL1 for people telling you to 'fuck off' for knocking on their door to sell them something they already had while interrupting an episode of Jeremy Kyle. The best I ever got was a cup of tea with an old lady who had a dog with one eye, and I got what was an easy sale because she felt sorry for how fucking wet I was.

Anyway, I'm not here to bore you with *Memoirs of a Door Knocker* by James Smith. To cut a long story short, one day, close to a breakdown, with my feet fucking freezing and a savage dead leg from rugby training the night before, I called my boss. I was done. I'd rather do bar work or go back to working as a labourer than this. At least when carrying bricks I was warm, could feel my feet and got told to fuck off less. Just about.

My manager told me to wait as he went to his computer. He then went on to say words that would change my perception for ever. He said, 'James, I have your stats here: every hundred doors you knock on, you eventually make a sale, that's your average. Some days you've made none, others up to five. So go knock on a hundred doors, mate. If you need two sales, then you'd best knock on two hundred …'

And it clicked for me right then – something I had never really thought about before. Everyone has averages to work with in all spheres of their lives. This doesn't just apply to doors, but everything.

You can be really bad at chatting up someone you find attractive, yet there will be a certain number of people you have to talk to before you get a phone number: for a seasoned expert in the field of dating it may be two numbers obtained from every four people spoken to at the bar; for someone less experienced it may take twenty different conversations with twenty different people to get just one phone number.

You can influence your average in every field you desire. It usually boils down to repetition and experience, but for me, with the doors, it would have been about how I dressed, how wet I was from my day's knocking or how much coffee I'd had. Some days, approaching a door with a dead leg or a black eye from rugby certainly didn't help my average.

So let this motivate you, not deflate you. Your ability to manipulate your average in every area of your life is controlled by you and your attitude, your ethos and your audacity. There are a certain number of interviews to attend and uncomfortable conversations to have with people in bars or even at the gym. Where your average is right now is not important, but what you do to positively affect that number is.

Just remember, whether that number is high or low, it doesn't change the fact that you need to do what you need to do. It's so often simply a case of getting that first awkward conversation or activity out of the way – a bit of a leap of faith – then, rest assured, it's all part of the numbers game. We are a walking and talking manifestation of our daily actions and habits. We are a physical representation of what we do each and every day. By taking control of these things we can construct who we are, how we act, what we look like, and how we feel.

Polarization – Your New Way to Be Intentionally Unpopular for a Better Life

Imagine if you invited me to a barbecue for your next birthday celebration. I'd come round and meet your family and friends, none of whom have met me before. I'd politely shake hands, make eye contact as I talked to people and thank the host for inviting me. Imagine I then sit down and sink a couple of beers and, a few minutes later, in an open discussion, I hear your uncle or someone talk about Formula 1. The conversation goes a bit quiet, the perfect opportunity for me to contribute. This is the first time I have ever met any of these people. What do I say?

'Formula 1 is awful! It's one of the most boring sports I've ever watched. Driving around different tracks, seeing who's the fastest, riveting. Cricket is a much better sport.'

All eyes are on me. There's an awkward silence. And then the next person will have their say. Now, not only have I remained true to my beliefs here, but at the same time I have cleverly polarized the entire group. (Lewis Hamilton, if you're reading this, I am sorry. Actually, no, I'm not. It is boring, mate.) By doing so, I have hopefully got at least 80 per cent of these guys to think I'm a bell end. But by doing so, I've brought the other 20 per cent – those who share my opinion – much closer. They might then think, Who is this guy? Who brought him along? I also fucking hate Formula 1 and I think I'm going to go grab another cold beer to find out more about him and what he does for a living.

A common perception or belief – especially in adults – is that we have enough friends. And when giving a business seminar, I've seen this trickle down to personal trainers trying to build a business: they might have enough followers, but they don't have enough *engaged* followers who become clients. For someone to convert from follower to client, and commit to buying from you, they need three things: to know you; to like you; to trust you.

So you're better off with 20 per cent of attendees at the barbecue loving you than 100 per cent of them not even remembering your name.

This is something I've been applying successfully for several years within the fitness industry. I am often crass, bold and sometimes come across like a prick, but I need to do so in order for the hypothetical 20 per cent to become closer to me, my brand, my ethos and my beliefs. People ask me how I deal with criticism and negativity, but little do they know I'm trying my hardest to *make* most people dislike me in order to make some people love me. **This, in turn, creates trust and a community of like-minded people**, which doesn't just mean success for me, but for my members too. Being unapologetically myself draws in those who are like me and repels those who are not, and means that when my members meet each other at events or spot each other in the gym, they have a lot in common (they all usually tend to swear as much as I do too).

For The James Smith Academy Pty Ltd hypothetically to make £1 million a year I need 9,259 people to commit to me for the 3 x Premium month block membership (which at the time of writing is only £108). In other words, to turn over £1 million a year, I only need

0.014 per cent of the UK population to like me enough to trust me to be their PT. I'm not trying to be a capitalist here or the next Grant Cardone, I'm just letting you know you can accomplish a huge amount without being hugely popular, and that trying to get everyone to love you is not only exhausting, it's also not smart.

If you get enough people to dislike you, you'll have another group who love you. Have you ever realized how exhausting it is not to be unapologetically yourself all the time? How it affects your mood and your headspace, having to conform to someone else's idea of what you should be like? A lot of my clients over the years have let a bit of my approach and attitude rub off on them – swearing a bit more when they feel like it, saying what they're thinking and saying no more often. Being unapologetically themselves, a little bit more every day. This is a massive contributor to creating the mindset you need for not only your success, but your mental health too.

Imagine from now on that you have a sieve in your life and only you decide who gets through it to spend time with you or do business with you. Every time someone walks into your life you shake that sieve; you find out who genuinely loves the unapologetic version of yourself *and who doesn't*. Some say we are the five people we spend the most time with, so make sure they are people who support you, challenge you, have your back, but most importantly aren't boring turds who want to watch cars do laps on a Sunday afternoon and call it a sport.

I'm known for never dressing very smart. I had to wear a suit when I worked in corporate and now you're lucky if you see me with shoes on. It's not that I don't care about my appearance, it's that I don't care about conforming to someone else's idea of what I should wear.

I've had very important, potential career-changing meetings with some very important people. I'll stand in reception usually in a pair of shorts and often with my skateboard in hand. (I like to skateboard, and my legs really get hot.) If someone doesn't like me, or the fact I skateboard around as a fully grown adult, then fuck them. I've not missed out on anything in particular – it's just a nugget stuck in the hypothetical sieve. We shouldn't change our identity for anyone, let alone for a false idealism that won't make us happy in the long run.

Bottom line: be yourself. It's exhausting if you're not. **And if you get enough people to dislike you, you'll be left with a new bunch of people who love you for who you really are.**

Effort and Ambition

I'm not here to lecture you, but this is important. Effort was a word I grew up hearing and seeing a lot, whether it was my mum's attempts to make me try harder at school or in the reports teachers would write: 'James needs to give more effort in class.'

Admittedly, I gave very little effort to most elements of my life until my mid- to late-twenties. I think passion is a spark that can ignite effort in any direction. This is why it's very important that we choose a career that is in line with what we love in life. What you love, your passion, is the direction of the wind, so kick with the wind because **life is too short to have a job you don't absolutely love**. I've become quite the quote-smith during this process, so I hope you're keeping a mental note of these to pull out in the future when you're staring down the barrel of making some life choices.

I didn't simply lack effort. I know that now. I work around ten to twelve hours a day. The main difference is that I now love my work, whereas before, I had no passion so I couldn't really give enough effort. But because of this, at school I was classified as having a learning difficulty. And it didn't take me long to realize that it was possible to trade my learning difficulties into a free MacBook in the months leading up to going to university if I was to attend an appointment with an educational psychologist. So I took a test with an educational psychologist, including odd tasks such as poking a pencil through different holes in a bit of card, and I left, rubbing my hands together at the prospect of a brand new laptop. The report concluded:

*'James has an above average IQ and an exceptionally fast
reading speed; your son does not have a learning difficulty,
he is just idle.'*

Random Educational Psychologist, c. 2009

I think that someone's ability to work hard is always there, you just need to find the connection to unlock it. The key to this is to put your efforts in the right places. Putting them in the wrong places and/or those that yield no return often brings about 'demotivation'.

If you consider that we are not so different from our ancestors, who had to spend days without food, hustling every day to quite simply not die, it's clear we have that drive inside us. We have a sympathetic nervous system, which gears us for fight or flight. Society has dimmed our ability to channel this, but it's something that practising Brazilian jiu jitsu (BJJ) has helped me to learn: should you need to, in the right situation, you can accomplish a hell of a lot … you just really have to need or want it enough.

Playing rugby for fifteen years was fantastic for me too, and I think that contact sports are great. Physical toughness goes hand in hand with mental toughness, there's no denying it. However, combat sports are a little different, and Brazilian jiu jitsu has been a game changer for me. Rather than getting on the field to see who can out-tactic their opponents through clever plays, it involves stepping on to a mat at a competition where there's only one gold medal.

To initiate the fight in sparring or competition you slap hands then bump fists to engage in the round. Once the fists touch, it's a fight. There's a lot of nerves I can't describe. In rugby you can make mistakes, miss tackles or not hear a certain call that's being made, and the game goes on, but in combat sports, one mistake can mean losing, which means that your two-hour journey to the competition, making weight and all the prep and training could be over in ten seconds, and you're going home with your tail between your legs and nothing to show for it in terms of silverware. Of course, lessons are always learned despite losing, but where the margins are so small it means you have to be extra switched on to prevent them. It's a mental challenge like no other; quite simply, one thing you may have learned at a session you weren't even going to go to can be the difference between winning and losing.

Anyone you know who has started a combat sport – whether it's boxing, kick boxing, BJJ or something else – will tell you about how healthy the mindset of fighting another human is – with rules, of course, so no one gets hurt. Conflict is something we've had to deal with for millions of years and it's in our DNA. To deny the emotions we feel in certain situations is not healthy. We need to let them out, and contact sports are amazing for this.

Social structures and employment hierarchies at times also affect the potential for much-needed conflict to play out, and I think having a sport like BJJ as a form of escapism can have a positive impact on how you deal with these situations. I also believe, from first-hand experience, as well as from my clients, that when someone learns to protect themselves physically it transfers mentally. Your attitude is physical and mental: we often separate the two, but I believe they're more closely aligned than we tend to acknowledge.

Everyone has a form of escapism. Unfortunately, for many it's alcohol and partying at weekends to dull the emotions around Monday approaching. Mondays don't suck, though. If you think they do, it's just that your job sucks in most cases. But knowing you can fight someone for a ten-minute round in front of dozens of people in BJJ, suddenly the prospect of handing in your notice and finding another job doesn't seem so daunting, right?

People seem to think they don't have what it takes to leave a job or a relationship, and often this is because of their limiting beliefs. These are certain beliefs we create inside our heads; I believe they're a protective mechanism, but we must discredit any that don't have evidence to back them up. One of my biggest limiting beliefs surrounded what I deemed people would pay me. There was no physical evidence or data that people wouldn't pay me more, so I increased my hourly PT rate, lost no clients and realized how false my limiting beliefs had been.

In BJJ, when you tie your belt, bow before entering the mat and shake hands, your job, your race, your beliefs and your political standpoints are not important. All that is important is the respect you and your opponent give to one another before and after you try to strangle each other as hard as you can or opt to pull their leg off.

There's a Portuguese word, *'porrada'*, that's used within the jiu jitsu community. Everyone in Brazil knows *porrada* and it means 'brawling'; I believe that's the literal translation, but everyone uses the word for training hard = *porrada*.

#EverydayPorrada *means being intense in all aspects of life. On and off the mats. It's not only about training hard, killing yourself every day on the mats, it goes beyond that. It is a lifestyle for tough people who don't complain and make things happen in all aspects of their lives.*

One of the best decisions I ever made was to start BJJ, and it's also been one of the most humbling experiences of my life.

It's a sport that is honestly for everyone, you'd be welcome at any academy worldwide, and I don't think you're ever too old to get involved or try something that's outside your comfort zone. There are five belts – white, blue, purple, brown and then black. It takes around two years to progress to each one with frequent training, and there are four stripes marked on your belt between each level to show how close you are to the next grading. I'm blue belt, and although I've competed at that level, I've found the entire experience incredibly challenging, including the fact I've had to make weight for competitions.

I'd say my first stripe on my white belt was one of the toughest mental challenges I've ever had. It could only be described as drowning. In terms of athletic prowess, I'd have backed myself against almost all of my opponents. However, they then folded all the clothes I had on while I conveniently remained in them. I was stronger, fitter and sometimes more able-bodied than my opponents, but they knew that and could easily dismantle my strength, and there was nothing I could do about it. I felt like human origami in my first ever session.

The intention is to take your opponent to the floor and submit them or muster enough points through taking positions to your advantage. You need to have a good idea of where your limbs have their limit and know when you're about to pass out. I have had fully grown men sit on my head, crush my ribs bend, my fingers and throw me to the floor as I'd be thrown into the mat. Luckily, apart from a few sore fingers and a sore neck, I have not sustained any real injuries due to the respect in the sport and the rules that protect you.

I can't tell you how many times I've fancied quitting. I'd travel twenty minutes to training, get beaten up for an hour then leave exhausted, frustrated and unable sometimes to even take my T-shirt off when I got home.

When I reached 100,000 followers on Facebook, we had a big party in Bondi to celebrate. The following week, I turned up to training and, as a white belt, I had the duty of wiping down the mats. It didn't matter how many followers I had or how successful I was in my business, I still hadn't earned my stripes to avoid wiping the mat down. But I loved every moment. The man next to me could be the CEO of a FTSE 100 business, a doctor or even a mechanic, and it meant nothing within the realms of how accomplished we were in the sport. It wasn't just humbling, it was great.

Since my first stripe, things haven't really got easier. I still have to attend and travel to training, and there is always someone better than me who will kick my arse. The effort put into the task of becoming a better BJJ athlete never stops. It never will either. The amount of struggle required in every session, every day is not to be ignored or overlooked. Since the initial stripe, I have taken so many lessons from the sport and applied them to life. We roll six- to ten-minute rounds; if you're submitted, you begin again. There is no escaping the time left. No matter how good your opponent, you're in it for the long haul, so you'd best be willing to struggle and give everything you have in every position.

There is also always going to be someone better than me. That's powerful when you think about it. I am at peace with that in my BJJ life, my work life and all aspects of my life. Who is better than me is not important. All that matters is what I get done with my daily struggles.

> *'Who you are is defined by what you're willing*
> *to struggle for.'*
>
> Mark Manson, author

I love the sport because it firmly connects me to the notion that there is nothing in front of my progress or ego except for my next stripe. I need to work and develop in every way I can for that; nothing else is important. To put this in context, if I had 20kg to lose in body fat and that 20kg was always at the front of my mind, it'd be like worrying about my black belt opponents when I'm still a white belt. There are days when I feel like I'm making progress, there are others when I get destroyed, I make mistakes, I feel like I have no energy. But as I've said already, what I tell my clients is to focus on that first kilogram and then we'll think about the next one. **Progression and development aren't linear** – not in BJJ and not in fat loss or training either; we can't expect to leave each day a little stronger and a little fitter. There are cycles of ups and downs, but what's important is to focus on our attitudes after those down days – we just need to wash our kit, go to bed and make sure that tomorrow is a new day with a new attitude to face the challenges that follow.

Aggression – the good kind

Every day, as well as effort, it's important to turn up with intent, with a goal, with a direction and with aggression too. Aggression isn't what happens when you have ten pints of beer and want a fight. It's a sensation that you can feel in your stomach of determination to get something done.

Aggression is what gets you out of bed when you're tired, it's the internal monologue you have as you look at yourself in the mirror in the gym. As a part of your brain tells you that no one will notice if you skip your last set of exercises, it's aggression that rises from the belly and tells you to harden the fuck up. The aggression isn't towards other people training – it's from you to you. It says let's do two more reps than planned and it takes your performance beyond the realms of what you considered possible before the set.

Aggression is required to step onto a gym floor you're anxious to go on; it's required to hit 'apply' on a job you saw online because you're sick of your existing set-up; and it's the same aggression that sends the text saying 'we need to talk' to your partner who's not fulfilling their part of the relationship.

Aggression is a key part of the 'get-shit-done' mentality, when you need to rev yourself up to overcome some very intimidating scenarios. You may be four sets away from the best workout of your life on the leg press, and you may need to muster that aggression to go over to the intimidating man and ask, 'How many sets have you got left?'

Something as trivial as a question to a stranger can have a very empowering effect, and you'd be surprised how that translates into other areas of your life. I read a book that said to look a stranger in the eye when walking past, and not break eye contact before they do. You'd be surprised at how liberating that exercise is in building your comfort zone. You can walk down a street and make little advances towards becoming the person you want to be and need to be in life with something as simple as not breaking eye contact.*

Not every day is going to be a good day with training, and you need to ensure your mindset is in the right place. Don't blame anyone for anything. That's where failure stems from. This isn't a blame game. When someone submits me in BJJ that's on me, not anyone else. I must look internally and decide where I grow, where I focus my efforts and what I can do to prevent it or better myself.

To conclude: you may not choose to partake in adult playfighting, but your attitude of everyday *porrada* can be used in the gym, work, working out or just everyday life, and it's essential to the 'good life' you strive for. You're harder than you give yourself credit for. We know sleep is essential for a good state of mind, but maybe having a fight with a friend or stranger with some rules there for everyone's safety could be

* Don't do this while sitting on the machine in the gym, opening your legs against resistance. It doesn't look good.

a fantastic addition not only to your training regime, but your perception of your own identity and abilities.

It is only from outside our comfort zone that we truly grow. **Remember that a ship is safest in harbour; however, that is not what ships are made for.**

Effort 2.0: The Beginning of 'Overnight Success' – Intention and Empowerment

Looking back at the tail end of 2016, I was struggling a bit with the direction my life was going in, and when I set off to Australia on a one-way ticket I had no idea what I was going to do. I left the UK with a backpack, a few-thousand pounds in savings and a couple of books. I figured that things would sort themselves out, and the worst-case scenario was that I could always move back in with my parents (which still appeals to me to this day, as my parents are quite simply the best, literally).

I had left the UK as a highly paid PT with a fully booked diary, but – for the second time in my life – **I had caught one of the worst diseases that can ever hit a human: boredom**. I was at a music festival in Croatia when, at about 3 a.m., I turned to my friends in the middle of the dance floor and said: 'I'm moving to Australia.' I was not sure how I drew that conclusion at that point in time, but I made my mind up there and then. I didn't think it was 'the right thing to do', but I knew it was what I needed to do.

Six weeks later, I was gone. Some of my clients cried when I told them I was going, and I certainly had a lump in my throat looking back at my time in a gym I'd spent three years in, notching up thousands of hours of PT experience, which laid the foundations for a journey much larger than I ever expected.

When I touched down in Cairns, Australia, I had a 2011 MacBook, a set of tangled Apple headphones, a couple of books and a bucketload of ambition. I travelled down the coast solo, riding Greyhound buses, to eventually find out that Sydney, Australia, was going to be the place I called home.

I had some online PT clients and I signed on as a self-employed trainer with Fitness First in the Sydney CBD, and for the first time in my life, I had to give maximum effort. I loved Australia and I still do. I could write a sequel to this book on just that alone. My drive was based purely on the fact that if my business did not perform well enough, I was going home to the UK, trading sunny Bondi days for Berkshire. Every walk on the beach would give me an internal reaffirmation of the work ethos I would need to remain there – and Australia is not cheap!

I was really not sure what my identity was going to look like within the Sydney PT scene. I was an outsider, a blond 'Pom' without a six-pack, no significant following on social media and not much more than a good attitude mixed with ambition and some audacity. Funnily enough, I couldn't afford to move into my own place, even when I joined Fitness First, so I was living in a hostel in the CBD – which I kept secret. My cashflow from online PT wasn't always the most consistent, so there were several days when I had to book three to four days of the dorm at a time, and then check out and check back in. I couldn't afford to book further ahead than that, so I had to sit in reception for a few hours up to twice a week. And I'd always queue a bit early so I could get a bottom bunk.

I had a lot of time on my hands, so one day, with my fresh new business PT Instagram page, I decided to identify the top ten gyms and PTs in the Sydney CBD. I then manually followed their followers one by one. This would take me hours on end each day – I nearly walked into so many lampposts. Over a period of a few weeks – on buses, in the reception of my hostel or walking by the beach – I followed 7,500 people. I figured that if 10 per cent followed back, I'd have 750 people following me in Sydney. If I could convert 5 per cent of those into clients, I'd have a full diary for PT. *That's quick maths.*

Effort should not be underestimated. I had to commute from Manly, where I moved after my time in the hostel, and I had to get the ferry into the Sydney CBD. But I never forgot to carry Tim Ferriss's book *Tools of Titans* with me. It helped me at a very challenging time through his concept of the gun-to-the-head mentality.

My internal dialogue went like this: 'I'm working as hard as I can day in, day out to accomplish what I want to.' But come to think about it, if you'd put a gun to my head and asked me again, I might just have called every single one of my online clients and not put the phone down until they gave me two referrals each. I could have given out fliers for my business on a nearby busy street to the gym where I was working. And in time this attitude has become habit for me, without needing to think about a gun to my head for me to do what I need to do to succeed at something.

We can always do more. I feel we just kid ourselves about it more than we realize. I'm not just talking business either – I'm talking about all the excuses we feed ourselves. Someone out there is having it tougher than you are, and they're outworking you right now in every area of life. They have the same hours on the same days, but their secret ingredient all along has been effort. To consider a gun to your head before you next feed yourself an excuse is a powerful tool to use, not just while you are reading this book, but tomorrow and every day when you are immersed in the struggle – which will be every day. And let's not forget that our *perception* of our daily tasks and struggles is also very important for us to achieve them.

Mark Manson said it brilliantly in *The Subtle Art of Not Giving a F*ck*, about a marathon. If you wake someone up, pull them out of bed and tell them they have to run 26 miles, it'd quite easily be one of the worst days of their life. However, give that person six months to get ready for it and a nice pair of shoes, and it could easily be the proudest day of their year or even their life. They may even get their parents to come and watch.

So how does all of this relate to diet and fitness? Putting it simply: if you're not happy in your career right now, and you're not happy with your home life – whether it's a toxic relationship or constant bickering – I know it's sad to admit, but eating could be the thing that brings you the most happiness in the day. Never forget that the common message thrown around in the industry – **'eat less, move more'** – **could be translated as: do less of what makes you happy (eating), then do more of what makes you unhappy (throwing yourself at workouts that bring you no enjoyment).** This isn't a good place to be in for sustainable dieting. You need a diet that doesn't feel like a diet and a workout regime that you look forward to. I honestly feel everyone will enjoy some form of training, but some people just don't try enough things to find it.

Goal setting

When I think of every cringeworthy pitch from any 'business-development guru', I always imagine them talking about goal setting. Setting real goals enables me to give the effort I need each day, and that's why I've put this section in the book just after effort.

In 2017, I had a PT mentor in Sydney and, against my will, I was made to write my first ever 'vision board'. My eyes rolled into the back of my head, as I thought this was some classic guru bullshit. The guy pulled out an A1 bit of paper – that's huge, by the way. I thought to myself several things. Firstly, Who the hell prints on A1 paper? Secondly, Why am I planning trivial shite when I could be napping?

I had to write down three goals for the year, a lifetime goal, books I was going to read and things I was going to accomplish. It was a ball ache. I then had to start breaking up the goals into stages of how I was going to accomplish them. For the first time, I had to actually think about how I would do it.

I set a lifetime goal of 100,000 followers on social media. The objective for 2017 was to reach 30,000. I randomly wrote that'd I'd like to host three seminars in two countries (UK and Australia) and that I'd like to earn $100,000 for the year. I wrote this in January.

Sounds sad to say it, but I stuck the A1 bastard on my wall at home and it was the only thing up there. My room was incredibly bare, and every time I turned my light on at 5.45 a.m. I had this ugly poster staring at me, reminding me about the books I was going to read and those seminars I had to give. I remember a moment very vividly when I had written down the salary I was aiming for, the $100,000 dollars. Month on month, I wrote down what I had earned and subtracted it from that total to keep me aware of how far I had to go.

Earning the money wasn't hugely important to me, but getting on my own two feet again was. Before I got to the vision board stage I've just described, I was travelling the East Coast and ran very low on money, to the point where my dad had to book me a flight home on Christmas Eve. He only found out at the last minute that I'd left it so late because I couldn't afford a flight.

On New Year's Eve, as the clock struck midnight, I was asleep at my parents' house because I couldn't afford to go out with my friends.

When I decided I wanted to move to Australia, I had to sell my Golf GTI and I lost about £1,400 selling it.

I still have the sticker in the first page of my passport from my 'Air China Experience'. I booked the cheapest flight I could find to go back to Sydney. I had a thirteen-hour stop-off in Beijing with no social media and no emails due to Chinese laws.

You can buy any Gucci handbag you like in Beijing airport, but you can't buy deodorant or toothpaste – the same stuff that got taken out of my washbag at Heathrow. I travelled for nearly forty hours without being able to reapply deodorant or brush my teeth. I didn't care at the time, I just wanted to be back in Australia. I got off my second flight, having watched *Saving Private Ryan* (in Chinese), and moved into my hostel for three nights before having to sit in reception to check in again for the next booking I could only just afford.

Once I was sharing a flat with my friends again, I came home one day to be left with the bill for all our stuff. Ben, my very good friend who at the time worked in PR but could easily have been an interior designer, pretty much kitted out the flat from IKEA. Again, at twenty-seven, I messaged my dad and asked to borrow a bit of money to pay for the sofa. That conversation stung me deep inside: my old man, without hesitation, sent me about £2,000. I felt a bit disgusted that I had been making a fair bit of money back in the UK, but had not really saved any of it and now my dad was paying the price. So when I set a financial target on my vision board, I assure you it was with one thing in mind: *to never have to borrow money from my parents again, ever.*

January was a pretty slow start. I began at Fitness First, and by March I remember marking the vision board with an impressive $12,200 figure for my online and face-to-face business combined. I sat back and thought to myself, James, this is good and if you do it again next month, you can pay your dad back before he thinks about charging interest.

Now, this is the part where the story comes together and my entire standpoint on vision boards changed for ever. April came to an end and I had to calculate what I had earned across both online and face-to-face. It was similar to before. I entered $12,100 on that paper on the wall. And it was only the act of physically writing down my earnings that made me realize I'd earned $100 less than the month before. I was mortified. I sat on the edge of my bed and felt like I was going backwards for the first time in my life.

I often ask myself whether, if that vision board had not been there, things would have been different. Anyway, the month of May started with me booking my first ever seminar. I didn't care how I was going to get people there, but it was time to start accomplishing some of the things on my vision board. I had the return leg from Air China booked for May either way. I never missed an alarm in May. No matter how cold it was, I went outside and did my Live videos, and I never missed a social-media posting window I'd set myself.

I flew home, and had nearly 200 people attending my seminar. I remember the twitch I got in my eye from being on my laptop so much. I returned to Australia exhausted, and I tell you what: *Saving Private Ryan* second time around in Chinese isn't as good as the first.

One day in June, I realized I hadn't entered May on my vision board. I ran a PayPal report, the earnings from the seminar and the very few face-to-face sessions I had done. I had to get my friend Lucy to check my calculations – I was sure I was wrong, I had to be wrong. In the month of May 2017, in a desperate attempt to ensure my earnings did not to decline further, I'd managed to earn $29,000. The impact of writing down April on my vision board had evolved into an attitude that I hadn't seen in myself before.

I paid my dad back, then thought about it and realized that with the money I could book a Sydney seminar, London and then Manchester again in the summer. I'd then have my international seminars ticked off my vision board list, be on my way to my annual target and I could actually accomplish what I had set out to do for the year. I could win my first vision board.

This leads me to another law I want you to be aware of from this point forward: **Parkinson's law holds that however much time you allocate to a task, it will take that long to complete.** Otherwise known as 'work expands so as to fill the time available for its completion'.

Setting myself the time each week, month and year to accomplish tasks meant that whatever action I did on a daily basis was now time sensitive. Funny how when you only have twenty-five minutes to work out you can end up sore for days. Alternatively, give yourself all day to tidy the house and nothing gets done.

By July 2017, I'd pulled my vision board off my wall. I screwed it into a ball and threw it in the bin because I had completed everything on it that I'd wanted to. Little did I know that only a couple of months later I'd also have reached my lifetime goal of 100,000 followers. I do wonder how much seeing those things on the wall contributed to my daily actions and habits. Remember, waking up on time or ensuring that you do something every day isn't that amazing in itself, but the return on all those small things over time is what makes the difference.

I kept my 2018 vision board a lot simpler and aimed for 500,000 followers across Facebook and Instagram, to swim 500m freestyle without stopping and to obtain my blue belt in Brazilian jiu jitsu. The followers goal was only partly in my control – you can't force people to follow you. The blue belt was almost all in my control, but again, you can't force your professor to give you a belt, you have to earn it. But the swimming was 100 per cent in my control.

Some days it was too cold and I didn't want to jump in Icebergs' pool; some days I was sore and I hurt from training; and there were days I felt flat, but in essence, I knew that I would not accomplish any of the goals without the daily action. In my first attempt at hitting 500m I swam 630m; my blue belt was awarded to me on 11 November; and I hit 500,000 followers three days before the end of 2018.

A vision board isn't just about writing down your goals; it's about making them real. It was important to me that they physically existed, not even on a notes section on my phone or as a background. They had to exist, on a board, on a wall. Somewhere that I could see them. I often envisaged the day I pulled the piece of paper off the wall: would I be accomplished or disappointed? At some point the vision board must be rewritten – you have either accomplished what you set out to or you haven't. **Your daily actions and the cumulative effect of sticking to them determine the net result.**

If you have a goal in mind, write it down, make it real. Then do what you have to do to make it happen.

The inevitable plateau

The definition of a plateau is 'a state of little or no change following a period of activity or progress'. A plateau is inevitable in every realm of life, whether it's fitness, relationships or work, and it's very important that we consciously acknowledge how big a role our egos can play in this. **We have all had periods in our life when we have had some form of success, but then at some point, we seem to fall off or flatten out on the curve of the success or achievement in question.**

> *'When success begins to slip from your fingers – for whatever reason – the response isn't to grip and claw so hard that you shatter it to pieces. It's to understand that you must work yourself back to the aspirational phase. You must get back to first principles and best practices.'*
>
> Ryan Holiday, *Ego Is the Enemy: The Fight to Master Our Greatest Opponent*

Ryan Holiday's book (see References, p.286) got me thinking about the ongoing story we tell ourselves about ourselves, in which we often miss out the times we got lucky, worked incredibly hard and had a tough time. When we listen to that story, we put more emphasis on simply how brilliant we are naturally, even at all the times we actually got lucky. We like the sound of that story a lot more, making it easier to repeat to ourselves.

The danger of this comes from believing our own story. Looking back on my own life, I could tell myself a story of how I went to Australia with a dream, made funny videos and how I'm a funny guy or that I'm charismatic. I could then attribute my success to maybe my looks, outgoingness and candid approach – and, let's not forget, flawless audacity. I could then assume my success was in line with posting hilarious, educational, empowering content every day without fail.

To believe this story would be the demise of my ongoing successes in life.

This is because I would be overlooking the key principles of how I really became one of the world's fastest-growing online personal trainers. The truth is: I got up just before 5 a.m. for nearly a year; I set up a tripod in public to answer questions for people every day via social media; and I was exhausted most days, running off an aspiration to do more with my work and a plethora of 7/11 $1 coffees.

I remember having to speak louder as the 5 a.m. carpet cleaners came around where I was sitting; I had fifty people watching me answer questions and I turned up every day. Weekends, hungover, I'd do the same. If I had too much work, I'd have to go LIVE at 9 a.m. in front of work colleagues who mocked me, laughed at me and pointed as I set up my tripod in a busy area. They didn't see what I saw. And they didn't like what I was doing – which was more than they were.

People would walk past me thinking, What is this guy doing? And I remember them staring at my screen. All day, every day I was hustling for something bigger and more than what I had before. I gained weight, I lost my mojo to train in the gym and I burned the candle at both ends for a long time. When I tell myself the real story, it's imperative that I listen to what really happened. **It wasn't brilliance. It was determination and setting three alarms to ensure I got out of bed.**

If I listen to my ego's idealized portrayal of how I gained relative success, I run the risk of not recognizing the real fundamental pillars of what got me that success in the first place. By doing so my ego could and would run me into the ground through narcissism and a sense of confusion, as I lost my grip on what I have built so far by no longer paying attention to what it was that built it in the first place.

So what does this mean for you? Chances are you could very well do the same. When you lose some weight, some fat, some measurements, and move in the right direction, you can very easily start to tell yourself a story:

'I'm good at dieting.'
This could mean less-frequent tracking, fewer portions measured or even more meals out, mindless snacking and thinking you're intuitive enough to make it work either way.

'I'm so good at smashing my workouts.'
Skipping the odd workout, taking the odd lie in over a workout, shaving a few sets off each day; thinking you've done enough or accomplished enough so far to not warrant quite so much effort going forward.

'I'm really good at my job; I can get so much done without having to try too hard.'
No longer aspiring to go higher, not grafting for a pay rise or promotion and even slacking with the notion that you can't lose your job or get fired because you've done so much already for the organization.

In all these circumstances, often the solution lies in going back to where the success began. I actually found myself doing this within my first year as a trainer. I was the busiest and best-paid PT, so what did I do because of that?

I stopped prospecting and walking the floor because I was busy. I stopped checking in with my clients over the weekend because my diary was full. Before I knew it, things had changed. I had half the hours I had before, and I had no idea why at the time. I was a good trainer – why was I no longer busy? Quite simply, because I had stopped doing the very things that enabled me to have a busy diary in the first place. I listened to my ego and assumed I was busy because I was a good PT.

It's important we don't listen to our egos when striving to push past plateaus.

> 'If you start believing in your greatness,
> it is the death of your creativity.'
>
> Ryan Holiday, *Ego Is the Enemy: The Fight to Master
> Our Greatest Opponent*

The takeaway here is that we can't always stop this from happening (and, as you know, I'm a firm believer in getting plump at Christmas), but we can identify when it occurs and get ourselves back on track. It's

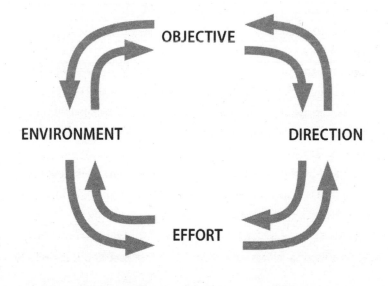

important to understand that who we are and how we act are not fixed, and even our internal communication with ourselves is very important. I want you to think about the analogy of the sailing ship: ships readjust their direction hundreds of times a second to remain on track. There's no such thing as sailing in a straight line. Should a ship not make seemingly small changes in direction, it would veer off course and potentially miss its destination by hundreds of miles.

Have I slipped away from the person I became before to get those results?

What principles, practices and attitudes do I need to re-adopt for progression to re-occur?

But it is not always attitude and ego that are to blame for discontinuation of results. Sometimes the culprit is within our physiology.

Dieting plateaus and metabolic adaptation

Metabolic adaptation is a real thing. It's all too possible that in a successful bout of dieting your components of energy expenditure have shrunk and small adaptations have occurred. If I were to diet on 1,500 calories, which is 50 per cent of what I've figured I need on a daily basis to be isocaloric (right in the middle, aka maintenance), eventually those 1,500 calories would stop working for fat loss. In the initial weeks, months, even years, I would lose fat, substantial amounts. With that I'd become lighter, therefore burning fewer calories when I move, which is a decrease in my NEAT (see p.63). Months of being in a calorie deficit would negate and impede my training performance and ability to exercise for long periods, which would affect my EAT component (see p.61). Quite simply, through eating less I'd reduce my thermic effect of food (TEF – see p.62) and being a lighter and smaller entity, this would influence and decrease my BMR (see p.60). All of these would help compile my total daily energy expenditure (TDEE) and, in turn, 1,500 calories – once a 50 per cent deficit – would be a 0 per cent deficit given enough time. *This is known as metabolic adaption.*

To conclude, when we find ourselves plateauing or slowing down, we need to assume it's not just our metabolism adapting, but perhaps our psychology, attitude and ethos too. Avoiding a plateau entirely is going to be difficult, so when it does occur, don't be deflated or disheartened – just get back on track to ensure that the small readjustments in attitude and approach are enough to keep you going until the next readjustment needs to occur. These adjustments are the small changes you make to your attitude and habits over time, whether it's reading more, exercising more or waking up at a different time.

Our internal dialogue is important too. Let's say I have a new client, Brittany, who tells me about her lifestyle, her sedentary job in a corporate office in London. The team she works with is huge and it's always someone's birthday. It feels like every day she's offered a cake, a tub of chocolate treats or even a glass of wine towards the weekend.

For years, Brittany has been yo-yo dieting and saying, 'I can't, I'm on a diet.' This language isn't great, as it insinuates that Brittany *does* eat those things – she loves them – but she can't because she has self-imposed a period of restriction, usually temporary.

Now, imagine if I was to get Brittany to fully believe that she's someone who doesn't have those kinds of foods during the week, or when she's at work. A new part of her identity. This internal dialogue calls for a huge amount of readjustment to the 'ship' of our attitude and ethos – not just to 'be on a diet', but to be a different person with a different identity. Your driving licence will look the same, your passport too, but who you are, what you believe and how you act tomorrow can be influenced – and will be influenced – when you put down this book today.

Impostor syndrome

Our ego sits on one side of the table, telling us how great we are, but for every narcissistic thought, there is usually an insecurity waiting in the wings, one of which is 'impostor syndrome'.

We all, at some point, will experience some form of success. It's worth noting that sometimes we may deem our levels of success rather insignificant when we compare our lives to others' on Instagram or television. But when we do experience any relative success or an opportunity arises, we can be left feeling like a bit of an impostor.

For me, this was most prevalent when I trained on the gym floor as a PT. Little did I know it was only the beginning of a long journey of feeling like a fraud. I nearly kept this subject out of the book entirely, but when I did a podcast about it earlier this year it was pretty crazy to hear how many people it had resonated with. So what exactly is it?

The term 'impostor syndrome' refers to a pattern of behaviour where people doubt their own accomplishments and have a persistent, often internalized fear of being exposed as a fraud.

Originally, it was thought to have been most prevalent in high-achieving women, but in researching the topic with friends and peers, I've found that it's something everyone deals with. This is the thing: I don't think it's quite possible to eradicate this notion of feeling like a fraud in our work; it's just something we have to consciously manage. I believe that impostor syndrome could easily fall into the same category as limiting beliefs (see p.142), and for this reason we need to pull apart the argument we create inside our heads as to why we could be thinking we're a fraud.

For instance, when I have an event where I need to speak in front of a thousand attendees, it's all too easy for me to think, Why are they here? Soon they'll find out I shouldn't be up on stage; it should be someone else, someone smarter, someone who can help them more. I then will have an internal monologue questioning this belief. Is it true? What do the facts state?

The facts would state it is not an accident that they're here. It's not an accident most things ever happen. Your job role, your next promotion, the next time you're asked to do something outside of your comfort zone: these are not accidents. I'm not sure if the impostor syndrome is there to protect us, to perhaps keep us grounded or living within certain limitations we believe about ourselves, but it's something you'll need to manage when moving on from this book.

Impostors on the gym floor – should I be here?

I think this occurs in a small way in the gym every day. For instance, when someone – especially a woman – wants to use the squat rack in a busy gym, their first thought is that they're not supposed to be there. 'Someone probably needs this more than me.' Their minds fill with thoughts of perhaps the PT who needs it more, someone doing a more complex lift, someone with more weight, and that they're not welcome in there.

Moving forward, we need to be pragmatic and dissect any limiting beliefs that are holding us back. I'd be lying if I said I didn't feel the pressure squatting in a new gym or new surroundings, so this is your best way of coming to terms with why you're welcome in that area of the gym. I'm surprised that the psychology of a squat rack hasn't been studied further!

You're not a fraud in here, go back to the squat rack.

Imagine this: you need to stimulate your body for your goal; one segment of this is your lower limbs. Ankles, knees, hips all need range of motion under resistance to ensure longevity of bone health, muscle health and joint health. You can use just your bodyweight; however, one day your body will not deem this enough for an optimal stimulus. You'll need to increase the stimulus (which I'll cover in more detail later in progressive overload – see p.257).

At some point, you will require more weight, then more weight again. Soon, the amount of weight you will require will surpass what you can physically hold on to. A barbell on the back is ergonomically the safest and easiest place to load that weight; you need a squat rack for safely loading and unloading between lifts.

That area of the gym is not reserved for muscular people or personal trainers, not for the gym-experienced folk or special people. Quite simply, it's there for someone who wants to load more weight than they can safely hold. Is that you? If so, **you're entitled to be there; you're not a fraud in any area of life and especially not in the squat rack**.

Any time you feel uncomfortable, out of place, unsure of whether or not you're an impostor somewhere, in a professional, social or training environment, just remember: it's normal to feel that way, you can't stop that, but you can manage it through picking apart the argument in your head; you're just telling yourself that bullshit so you don't have to worry about being intimidated.

Homework for you, from me: next time you're in a gym, and you see a squat rack – go use it, own it and enjoy it.

For tutorials on how to squat and all other gym movements visit www.jamessmithacademy.com

So I feel like the foundations have been successfully set in the first part of this book, and I want to progress and build on them in the second part. Things are going to get a bit more complex and interesting, but with each section completed, you'll become more knowledgeable and confident.

PART II
BUILDING ON YOUR FOUNDATIONS

Somatotypes and Sport Selection – Why You Don't Need a New Diet

I begin Part 2 of the book with something you probably wouldn't expect me to say to you. Something that may even shock you. The simple truth is: you do not need a diet; you already have one.

Now, depending on a few things, I can assume it may not be serving you as you want or would expect it to. For instance, if you're carrying more fat than you'd like, I'm afraid your diet contains too many calories for the amount you move. Should the opposite be the case – i.e. you seek weight gain – then I can tell you that your diet does not contain adequate calories. That's thermodynamics – oversimplified, of course. But fundamentally, that's the truth that a lot of people dance around when talking about dieting.

Over the years, people have thrown around different diets for this benefit and that benefit. Not only that, they have insinuated that there is even a diet for a certain 'body type'. So straight away your thoughts are derailed from what we've known for a long time about energy in vs energy out, and you're led on to a new path of thinking Okay, of course, it must be HOW I am eating, not HOW MUCH I am eating.

The three main and most often mentioned body types are referred to as mesomorph, endomorph and ectomorph – collectively known as somatotypes. These are very popular in advertising on social media. Keep in mind that communicating on social media is like talking to people who are in another conversation already, so you need something snappy to pull their attention away from what they're doing. 'Body type' propaganda is one of the most popular of these, I'd say.

American psychologist William Sheldon developed a concept in the 1940s whereby he categorized the human physique into three fundamental elements, which he termed 'somatotypes'.

Let's begin with a **mesomorph**, which is typically what you'd consider an ideal physique by societal norms: a good balance of muscle without too much fat (imagine 'meso' as 'middle'). Then, to the left, imagine an **ectomorph**, usually classified as tall and slim – someone who struggles to gain fat or muscle. Finally, there's **endomorph** (think 'end' – end of the spectrum, left to right). An endomorph gains muscle easily, but also fat, so they're usually of a thicker physique, let's say.

There's been speculation about having the right macronutrient split for your 'body type' in mainstream media, but I'd like to let you know these are not physiological but personality traits. Boom, mind blown.

BODY TYPES

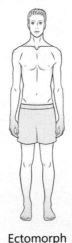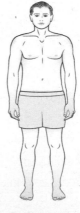

Ectomorph   Mesomorph   Endomorph

Psychology has been turned into physiology to get you to click on an advert.

I'd potentially make assumptions based on someone's body type, but I would never let it define them or what they're able to accomplish. For instance, let's say I have a consultation with Dave. He walks into the gym, I notice he's six foot four and very slim. I may start to theorise that perhaps his physiology has a part to play in his slim physique, but this is just a theory; it could also be partly to do with his psychology. Should Dave demonstrate mannerisms that could lead me to believe he's slightly anxious, I might conclude before I've even shaken his hand that he has a fairly low appetite (typically, I've noticed people who come across as a bit anxious tend to eat less than others), consciously or not. It's then for me, the coach, to talk to him about his eating habits and to ask if he sometimes forgets a meal. You become almost like a Sherlock Holmes as a PT, and you need to find out all sorts about your clients.

We all have slim friends who could fit into the category of the 'ecto' somatotype, and we notice they always eat whatever they like when we have meals with them.

Dave eats burgers and chips all the time, but still manages to stay so slim.

I've found over the years that people are vastly different in their eating habits and psychology. The same people who can get away with what we perceive to be a very calorie-dense diet often forget to eat. Someone like myself can't even comprehend what it would be like to forget a meal. I think about food from the second I wake up to the second I go to bed. That's arguably a psychological differentiator, not a physiological one, if you think about it.

Height also plays a role: the longer someone's levers are, the more space there is for muscle tissue to fill. Imagine, if you will, a beach with 250 deck chairs on it. Now, a big beach with 250 deck chairs may look desolate, but a small, secluded beach may seem busy and cramped with that many chairs on it. The point I am making is that sometimes muscle appears to be larger or denser on smaller levers – those who are vertically challenged, for instance.

So being six foot four, Dave has long levers, and therefore needs many metaphorical deck chairs to fill his metaphorical beach. Dave may also forget to eat for large parts of his day, so when I ask him his goal and he says, 'I want to gain a bit of muscle,' I need to be ready not to just say to him, 'Eat more.' I need a strategy in place to work alongside his current eating habits – something as simple as an alarm on his phone reminding him to eat or drink is so simple, yet so powerful.

Let's also not rule out that Dave may turn over nutrients very fast and have a faster 'metabolism' than most. So we're looking at long levers, a small appetite, and a one-size-fits-all plan just won't cut it here.

Metabolisms and 'body types' – the misconceptions explained

Metabolism is the chemical processes that occur within a living organism in order to maintain life.

I know that's not the sexiest definition for metabolism, but it's important to note that people do differ huge amounts naturally, not only in the amount of calories they burn a day, but in the speed with which they lose and gain fat. So although the mechanisms and principles (calorie deficit), remain the same, chances are that people will always differ individually with how fast they occur.

Unless your scooter is called 'metabolism', you don't need to kickstart anything.

I came across a study a few years ago, involving prison inmates who were told that if they gained a certain amount of fat within a certain period of time, they'd be released early from prison. As you can imagine, the inmates stuffed their faces with as much as physically possible, whenever possible, yet the differences in weight gain hugely varied from person to person.

Even with identical twins there are differences in fat and weight gain when following the same hypercaloric* diet.

So now let's look at the mesomorph. People are quick to point the finger to superior genetics and the elusive and much sought-after 'fast metabolism'; however, as coaches we must look past feeding our confirmation bias on how that person has obtained their physique. It's again important to note habits that can be a much larger contributor to the 'body type', rather than jumping to conclusions about how quick they turn over or metabolize nutrients.

I have noted that former clients, friends and even relatives that would fit the 'meso' somatotype usually eat more slowly than other people at the table. I watch how fast people eat (it's quite easy because I'm usually done first as a very fast eater myself). I could tell you the speed all my friends eat at, actually.

Ben Carpenter, who is another UK-based PT and a good friend of mine, first brought this to my attention in a post where he presented

* Hyper = too many (calories).

data on how increasing the number of times you chew your food can decrease food intake. (Ben, I'd say, is best known for breaking down scientific literature for everyday fitness enthusiasts to understand easily.)

In one study, chewing each mouthful forty times decreased intake by 11.9 per cent versus chewing fifteen times in both lean and obese subjects. However, we should also take into consideration that it may not be the chewing itself but the type of meal taking longer to eat in some cases. Foods requiring less time to eat may encourage greater consumption, for instance softer meals that require less chewing.

I know that 11.9 per cent doesn't exactly make you want to count to forty between mouthfuls in your next meal. But considering a sensible calorie deficit is usually a reduction of 15–25 per cent of someone's TDEE as a ball-park figure, it could make a substantial difference for someone who may not want to track what they eat or calorie count. Perhaps to be considered a tool for the tool belt when needed.

I know these things seem trivial, and they're by no means gospel, but think about what we've covered so far in this book: more sleep, tracking your NEAT, potentially being more mindful when eating or even eating slower, let alone not being so misinformed by zealots with their own agenda. So many tools on your belt to use for a better life. And we haven't even started on the nitty gritty of what you have considered 'dieting'.

At the end of the scale, we have the 'endomorph', which sounds like a form of Power Ranger, to be honest. The attributes of the 'endo' soma-totype would suggest that this person gains muscle easily, but also gains fat easily. The majority of humans in general are predisposed to gain fat fairly easily. I'd say that from an evolutionary standpoint alone it wouldn't make sense for us not to. I think it's important to note too that statistically, there are more people who gain weight easily than remain lean all year round without effort. And although it's unlikely, if we were to head into a famine in the next few months, the lean (and lucky bastards, metabolically speaking) would die first of starvation.

Life is too short to spend it continually trying to be the leanest you can physically be. There's a sweet spot, also known as balance; and I wonder about people who are obsessed about having a six-pack all year round when you think about how many hours of the day it is visible. Is there a significant enough return on investment to have such a low body-fat percentage?

Imagine someone who has assigned themselves as an 'endomorph' walks into the consultation. I don't think to myself, Ah, classic endo, and reach for my 'endomorph training programme'. Instead, it's quite clear – depending on how much body fat that person has – that they are consuming too many calories for the amount they move on a daily basis. Either that or they're converting sunlight into calories in some form of photosynthesis, which is just not possible.

The important thing here to realize and note is that it's not often that ectomorph or mesomorph body types are targeted for propaganda in dieting and fitness. The overweight and the obese are typically the most desperate for a quick fix, and some clever marketing message comes up saying: *Are you eating right for your body type?* This is a loaded question and it straight away gives the person in question the thought that they are not eating right for their body type. That must be it, they think. Ah-ha! It's not the fact that I consume too many calories; it must be my body type and the fact I'm not eating right for it. Consequently, energy balance – the key founding principle of fat loss – is not only overlooked, it's completely disregarded.

There are training considerations for people of different physiological compositions. For instance, I find my taller clients (lanky bastards) are much more comfortable doing sumo deadlifts over the traditional set-up because their femurs (thigh bones) are so bloody long. However, on the diet side of things, not only is your body type largely bollocks, the nutritional interventions that are sold or claim to be of benefit are just marketing gimmicks. Trust me. The main thing they're looking to get from you is an email address – it's classic marketing 101. People will do or say whatever they can to keep the cost of acquiring that email address as low as possible.

Do we pick our sport?

I'm just over six foot (I can't quite call myself six foot one, but I feel that six foot doesn't quite do me justice; thank the Lord I wasn't one inch shorter or I'd be five foot eleven, on the cusp of six foot, and no one wants that kind of uncertainty in life). I fluctuate between 92 and 96kg, seasonally almost. If I need to make weight for Brazilian jiu jitsu (BJJ), I need to get to 91kg. Christmas, holidays or periods when I'm writing a book, I will usually be more sedentary and, to be quite honest, if I don't need to diet, I won't.

At that weight, for my height I'm pretty dense – according to my last DEXA scan my bone density is nearly off the charts and, touch wood, I haven't broken a bone since puberty. If someone was to look at me in a line-up, they would straight away think I'm a rugby player. I played for fifteen years, back row, which means my job was to run into people fairly hard, tackle anyone running hard towards me and stick my head in places the pretty boys wouldn't. Now, here's the interesting part: people will think I'm broad and dense because I played rugby, but in fact, it's the other way round. **I played rugby because of my physique.**

You don't pick your sport, your sport picks you.

People aren't tall because they play basketball; typically, the taller players excel being closer to the basket and having longer reach and ability to pass and catch at a greater height. Long-distance runners generally have long legs and short torsos. Swimmers often are tall and the opposite of that, with long torsos and shorter legs.

As you'll start to realize, in some cases the athlete works hard to develop their skill for their sport, but a lot of the time they will kick with the wind of their genetics, height, weight, etc. As already discussed, some people are naturally able to remain more lean than others. Although again, a huge amount of this is down to habits, we still need to take into account the genetic phenomenon here and there.

What I find unfortunate is that if we see personal training as a sport, I can't help but feel that we're falling for the same misconception that we look the way we do *because* of our sport. We don't. And being in good shape and looking good without a top on are not good enough credentials for a fairly complex profession that has the ability to turn the quality of lives around.

Those who have the potential to change lives can qualify with an online course for a few-thousand pounds and a few hours of spare time. I think we need to question whether people are in the profession because they want to change the direction of the obesity epidemic and to help people live better quality lives.

Or they've ended up in the profession due to the fact that they're in good shape.

Not to say trainers in good shape can't be great PTs. But what if I told you I was hiring for a job?

Job Requirements:
Communication, empathy, knowledge, attentiveness, ability to run a self-employed business model. Must market themselves well, run an entire social-media strategy and understand PR.

Hours: 6 a.m. to 7 p.m., three lunch breaks and between five–nine one-to-one meetings each day.

(These are the unfortunate hours of a self-employed PT.) I get ten applicants. They come in. Can you imagine if I asked them all to take their clothes off and picked the one in best shape? If that's the criterion for finding the best possible trainer, stop the world, I'm getting off here.

I recently trained at a gym in South-west London and, upon checking the Personal Trainer board, I counted that over 80 per cent of the trainers had their tops off in their chosen display photo. They'd chosen that as their picture to market themselves as a coach. We don't pick our doctor, nurse, physio or driving instructors on how they look with their tops off. I just think it's a shame we select our personal trainer on those credentials.

Fitness Fallacies*

In this section of the book, I want to dispel many common beliefs that you've probably been led to believe in your life so far. This will be like your bible – refer to it any time a charlatan or zealot tries to convince you to believe in one of their fallacies. With every word you read here, you'll become less vulnerable to the bullshit. If they keep on chatting rubbish, just feel free to throw the actual book at them – it's why I opted to publish it in hardback.

Just before we get going, I want to make you aware that beliefs are everywhere and they influence you every day, even if you're not religious. If you have been wrong about any of the fallacies I'm about to talk about, please realize **I was wrong about most of these before too**.

The reason human beings have evolved so far beyond other species and animals is our ability to tell stories and get others to believe them. This is something I learned from Yuval Noah Harari's trilogy of books – *Sapiens*, *Homo Deus* and *21 Lessons for the 21st Century* (see References, p.286).

It's incredibly difficult to get 10,000 people to go to war unless they all believe in the same story. A man in the sky who made up commandments or an afterlife with a mansion for all your friends – whatever it is, it's all based around people's beliefs. To believe in something, whether it's true or false, is human nature, **so don't beat yourself up about anything you learn in the following chapters**.

---

* Fallacy: a mistaken belief, especially one based on unsound arguments.

As you read on, you'll hopefully understand a bit better why so many people not only succumb to these fallacies, but why they have such strong beliefs that they make the fallacy their life's work.

Starvation mode – does eating too little stop you from losing fat?

The concept of starvation mode is that if you do not consume enough calories, you will not only hinder fat loss, but you could possibly gain some back. A mainstream theory is that your body has a self-preservation mode when you diet too extremely, consuming too few calories, and that is the cause for a lot of people struggling to lose fat.

Starvation mode, I'm sad to say, is actually not really 'a thing'. Our wonderful bodies are capable of amazing things, but this mode is not one of them. Something to consider is *adaptive thermogenesis, also known as metabolic adaptation*. Now, I know this sounds complicated, but let me break it down:

- ► Adaptive thermogenesis = adapting to production of heat.
- ► Metabolic adaptation* = amount of chemical processes adapting.

Both terms are alluding to change in output. When we reach a traffic light our car's requirement for energy output is reduced to idle. You could call this a motor vehicle's adaptation to not needing to produce or burn as much fuel, as the car is not required to move at this point.

---

* We've already talked about this in Part 1, but let's take another look at it now in the context of starvation mode.

Pressing the accelerator would signify an upregulation in engine output to allow the car to generate movement. The amount of fuel a car uses is dependent on the demands of the driver and the capacity of the vehicle at the time.

Larger people typically burn more calories, therefore energy expenditure declines as people lose weight successfully. If we recall the components of energy expenditure from p.60, we have our BMR making up our resting elements of calories burned. Then, in the non-resting elements, we have our thermic effect of feeding, EAT and NEAT, representing workouts and non-planned movement.

Here's TDEE again from Part 1 to refresh your memory on what our energy expenditure on a training day looks like:

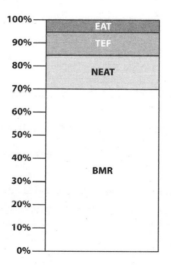

Does our BMR decrease through dieting? Is this what's going on during periods of 'starvation', also known as dieting?

'In weight loss, TDEE [total daily energy expenditure] has been consist-ently shown to decrease.

'Weight loss results in a loss of metabolically active tissue (such as fat) and therefore decreases BMR.

'Previous literature refers to this excessive drop in TDEE as adaptive thermogenesis, and suggests that it functions to promote the restoration of baseline body weight. Adaptive thermogenesis may help to partially explain the increasing difficulty experienced when weight loss plateaus despite low caloric intake.'

This pretty much means that there is a reaction from the body to spend less energy. Imagine, if you will, that you got a pay cut or you lost a few clients. Would that impact on your spending habits? Probably, yes: you'd make adaptations to ensure you didn't run out of money. In summary, TDEE can decrease as a result of adaptive thermogenesis.

'Exercise activity thermogenesis (EAT) also drops in response to weight loss. In activity that involves locomotion, it is clear that reduced body mass will reduce the energy needed to complete a given amount of activity.'

This means you'd burn fewer calories when training. This could be from being a lighter, smaller person performing an exercise or even from a drop in performance through not being as well fed as before.

If you're consuming less food in general, protein or other macronutrients, the body produces less heat in digestion and breaking down food. **A calorie deficit of any kind would decrease TEF; a calorie deficit paired with a higher constituent of protein would help prevent this from happening.**

'NEAT, or energy expended during "non-exercise" movement, such as fidgeting or normal daily activities, also decreases with an energy deficit. (…) Persistent suppression of NEAT may contribute to weight regain in the post-diet period.' (See References, p.286.)

This means you'd move less outside of the gym, whether it be an inclination to sit when the opportunity presents itself or to park closer to the shops. I covered this briefly in the fitness trackers part of the book (see p.67).

So the scientific literature backs alterations (usually decreases) in our expenditure of energy in periods of dieting, but what does this mean? It means that you may 'diet' on 2,400 calories, and yes, it works for a while. It then slows down to the speed of barely noticeable. This is because you're becoming a lighter, subconsciously less active version of yourself that has less food to digest each day. Eventually, you do not enter starvation mode; **the mode at play here is, simply, that your deficit calories are no longer a deficit**.

I found a study that found that successful weight-loss maintainers had a significantly higher step count than people at a similar body weight who had not lost any weight, suggesting that high physical activity could be a habit for successful weight-loss maintenance. (See References p.286.)

Adding this all together, it makes sense to emphasize the importance of keeping your activity levels high to offset any decrease in physical activity that can occur during periods of caloric restriction. Also known as keeping your #NEATUP247.

Starvation mode, as you can start to see, isn't something that makes any sense. However, I have several theories as to how it has come about as a common concept among fitness 'professionals'.

Scenario 1

A personal trainer doesn't want their client to get too excited and try to seek unrealistically fast fat loss when they're educated about a calorie deficit. They're told that the less they eat, the faster they'll lose fat.

So, the client in question could be planning something unsustainable in their head along the lines of vast reductions to their calorie intake: two Ryvita crackers a day and one bite of an apple for every gym visit.

The trainer, in a bid to protect their client from such a foolish move, tells a lie to his client: 'Don't drop your calories too low or your body will think you're starving and you'll gain fat!'

It makes perfect sense that someone would want to do that. There's psychological terminology called 'the hot-cold empathy gap', which is a cognitive bias where people underestimate the influences on their own attitudes, behaviours and preferences.

The idea behind it is that human understanding is state-dependant. When you're angry it's hard to understand what it's like to be calm, when you're calm it's vice versa. **People can succumb to this bias by setting goals for the future that are too restrictive** – it may seem like a good idea now, but that's because you're not experiencing how it feels to cut calories too low and be hungry. A short-term example would be when you set a really early alarm to go for a run as part of your new fitness regime, and it's only when the alarm goes off at 5 a.m. the next day that you realize you have over-estimated your enthusiasm, in the reality of that moment so early in the morning. It's been a battle over the years with some clients I have worked with to convince them not to try to fly out the gates too fast when it comes to calorie restricting.

Scenario 2

A newly qualified dietitian sets a calorie amount for their client Dave. Dave doesn't hit his calorie targets, not even close. The Cricket World Cup is on and the last thing he wants to do is get moaned at for being on the beer all weekend, so he responds to his dietitian: 'Yeah, hitting my calories, but no change in the scales, mate,' as he grabs another six-pack. After twelve weeks, he's actually gained a couple of pounds, and the dietitian concludes that he must be gaining weight because his calories are 'too low'. For some dieticians and trainers they'd rather believe someone was defying the laws of thermodynamics than that someone could just not be adhering to what they've been set.

To conclude, don't be fooled by anyone spouting nonsense about 'starvation mode'. Instead, educate them on what the science says about adaptation to new amounts of calorie intake. You're not going to store fat in a deficit, after all ... It's a deficit.

Overtraining

'Overtraining' is something that I get questioned about very regularly. People ask me if it exists – is it really 'a thing'?

Of course it is. In essence, all we're really asking ourselves is: 'Is it possible to overdo it?' In this case, **it's not just about our training, but more about our recovery from training**.

For instance, if we were to look at muscle stimulation as emptying a bucket of water, there are varying degrees of how much you could empty it. We look at recovery as refilling the bucket adequately and properly before the next pour.

So what would be ideal is if people saw the concept of overtraining as an issue of under-recovering – emptying the bucket before it has had the opportunity to fully refill – so that their response to the stimulus of training is then limited.

There is only so much exercise you can recover from in a week.

Now, the type of exercise, whether it be running, swimming, cycling, weight training, CrossFit, rugby or even a combination of all of those, will have an impact on how you can recover. Not only that, but we also have to look at the person recovering and what I could call '**internal variables**', such as age, gender, environment, genetics, as well as '**external variables**', such as sleep, nutrition, stress and hydration, to name a few.

All of these will fluctuate, especially the external variables. Your work schedule could get busy, warm weather has a negative effect on your sleep quality, your children have time off school or you get ill. A combination of several can hit you at the same time, and that can influence what you are able to recover from in any given period, such as a week. You may do three weight sessions a week, where you perform twenty sets at a good intensity. You may also run twice a week and swim once. Should a cold or illness of some kind come along, long hours at work or travel get in the way, it's optimistic for most people to keep up that level of frequency or intensity. Chances are you won't be able to recover from that amount of exercise, and it's good practice to taper it back. It takes trial and error, and a lot of the time people are frustrated by not exercising, whether they are an enthusiastic dieter or competitive athlete.

Elite athletes can often misjudge whether or not they're overtraining to get in shape, especially fighters. You can imagine the mentality of someone who is willing to go into a cage to fight someone in the UFC. They could have a runny nose or feel fatigued, yet they may decide to push through, despite their body giving them cues not to train. (There is also the external stress of knowing their opponent may train when they're resting.) And this is why it can be common practice for coaches across all levels to monitor their athletes' heart rate variability (HRV).

The reason I'm mentioning HRV is to highlight that even people at the highest level of sport aren't aware they're not fully recovering or adapting to their training. So don't beat yourself up that you're potentially overtraining without knowing it. Now, here's the sciencey part.

Heart rate variability is sensitive to changes in autonomic nervous system activity (i.e. changes in the sympathetic and parasympathetic nervous systems) **associated with stress**.

Think of **para**sympathetic as a parachute – a parachute slows you down. This is your 'rest and digest' part of the autonomic nervous system, and it's responsible for slowing the heart rate and a myriad of other roles in the body we don't need to get into here.

Sympathetic is the opposite – known as 'fight or flight'. We're supposed to be able to utilize both when appropriate, and in everyday life people can spend too much time in the sympathetic state because they have too much going on, contributing to stress. This is a contributor to poor recovery.

I don't think any of you will need to – nor should you really feel like – measuring your own heart rate variability, but I wanted to bring to your attention measuring stress. It's important for coaches to work with their athletes to minimize stress (outside of training) where possible.

It's worth noting that exercise to the body is stress. Living with a sixty-hour work week and then smashing yourself in the gym often makes things worse, not better. If Mike, corporate warrior who gets into the office at 7 a.m. and leaves at 7 p.m., realizes he's stressed and then joins a running club, he's still a sixty-hour-a-week stressed-out corporate, just with sore feet and a couple of blisters to add on top of it.

For Mike, the solution would lie within addressing the cause of the stress – i.e. his work environment – not just adding exercise to the equation and expecting it to deliver a magic solution. I once heard a bodybuilder talk on a podcast, and he said he found that a slight alteration to his regime, whereby he had the same working day but a slightly different commute, changed how much he could recover from in a week and he had to adjust accordingly. He even mentioned that something as seemingly insignificant as the slight anxiety of worrying about missing his stop on the train and being late for work each day had an effect on what he could recover from week on week.

For us to assume that our life environment does not vastly affect the amount of training we can each recover from each week is, I feel slightly naive, and it's very important we do our best to take readings from our bodies – **but not with our heart rates**, as I find that can be like using a sledgehammer to put in a nail. My own personal method is this:

'How tired am I out of 10?'
'How much do I want to train out of 10?'
1 2 3 4 5 6 7 8 9 10
Okay, should it be a 6 or below, I need to ask myself, 'Why?'

If we're motivated and we want something, we should always aim for the higher end of the scale. I'm a firm believer that no one wants to be overweight, obese, untrained or unfit. Now, our internal monologue here is very important: it's not a case of blame – saying, 'You don't want it enough'; we need a much more empathetic approach here:

'Why do I not feel so motivated to train?'
In almost all cases this will be due to:
- ▸ a lack of good-quality sleep
- ▸ a lack of sufficient nutrition
- ▸ stress-related fatigue
- ▸ being too tired from training

The last point here is the most important. Most people who are out of shape go through cyclical bouts of being ON or OFF with their diet and training. Getting back into them requires a bit of thought and being sensible. Going from no training sessions to three times a week can be very taxing to the body, and we need to empathise with ourselves when our bodies quite simply cannot handle the 'more is better' mentality – because it's not.

As well as being careful not to give our bodies too much to handle as far as output goes, we need to consider the input. The two biggest issues are these: firstly, the majority of people getting back into 'it' are dieting on a caloric deficit. Finishing each day with insufficient energy is not a great environment for recovery.

Another issue is the difficulties that normal people face for hitting adequate protein levels in their diets. The government guidelines are far too low, and to create and maintain an optimal environment for recovery we need more.

If we look at the science, what we have just been discussing is actually called 'over-reaching', while typically, a diagnosis of 'overtraining' can be considered diminished performance that lasts over months.

Technical overtraining = rare

Technical over-reaching = common

However, both are typically intertwined. According to research: 'Overtraining Syndrome [OTS] is a rare entity in the realm of over-reaching in which 1) excessive exercise is not properly matched with recovery and 2) an excessive stressor leads to significant mood disruption in the setting of maladaptive* physiology.' (See References, p.286.)

Now, I know you're not planning to do the next Tour de France, but there is no reason why you should not treat yourself like an athlete. If an athlete burns out, their performance will be hindered and they may let down some sponsors and not do so well in a race or event. However, if you burn out it could be the difference between you sticking to your diet and exercise regime and throwing in the towel because you find it too hard. Being tired, run down and deflated will not only have an impact on your training, but your family life, relationships and general

---

* Maladaptive: not adjusting adequately or appropriately to the environment or situation.

day-to-day activities too, and I need to ensure you don't overdo it and fall off the wagon at all.

Why? Because fitting into the clothes you want to wear for that next special occasion, whether or not you sustain it until your next holiday or make progressions you have never made before, could all boil down to your attitude towards your training.

I want you to think about three scenarios with me for a second.

1. What are the repercussions of doing too much vs not enough?

If you do too much – well, welcome to feeling deflated, flat, lacking motivation, poor mood, fatigue, decreased performance and a myriad other symptoms. But if you skip a gym session for an early night and wake up thinking, Do you know what? I actually feel fine, then you can go into the gym better rested, in a better mood and perform even better too.

Remember that it's only around 10 per cent of your daily calories within the EAT component. So, if you're tired or unsure, rest. Yes, I know, me the fitness and fat-loss guy is telling you to skip the gym, but better that than force a workout that leads you down a road of feeling super-tired and deflated – you have a life and profession outside of training, and although I want you to think like an athlete, you need to protect your energy at the same time.

Ever heard anyone say, 'The only bad workout is the one you miss'? Well, what a load of bollocks that is. Don't be falling for it.

2. What are the repercussions of returning to training too early vs too late after an injury?

Let's say you develop some form of niggle or injury, and you're advised to take three weeks off. You're impatient, you're eager to progress, you don't want to lose what you've worked so hard for. So you hear the physio say three weeks, but you go back in two. What are the implications of this? *If you do the same injury again that's another three weeks.* If it's worse than the initial one – which is very possible – it's even longer. Your impatience could then cause you to be staring down the barrel of six weeks now rather than three.

On the flip side, what if you took a week longer than you were advised? You'd go back to training with a much lower risk of re-injury. It's very important to consider these things and weigh up the repercussions of both scenarios. Sure, it's another week, but you could be saving yourself weeks of time off in the long run. You could even perhaps work some very easy rehab stuff in that extra time.

3. What are the repercussions of not hitting your daily protein target vs overshooting it?

Daily protein can seem like an absolute ball ache from time to time, but it's essential as part of the environment you need to create for optimal recovery. Should you be too low, you can remain in something known as a 'negative protein balance': 'When faced with a decrease in dietary protein intake, the body will adapt. However, if protein intake is inadequate the body will not fully adapt but will enter a state of accommodation that is characterized **by a reduction in physiologic functions**. For example, older women who consumed 56 per cent of the recommended daily allowance for protein for 10 weeks experienced profound reductions in lean body mass (2–5 per cent decrease.' (See References, p.286.)

A lot of people talk about 'too much protein', and there are one of two reasons why this notion has made it into mainstream talk:

1. Gluconeogenesis .

If the body needs carbohydrates and has more protein than it needs, it can convert protein to carbohydrate with this process. It's worth noting this very rarely happens, but all too often, people who are poorly educated in the subject will proclaim: 'Don't eat too much protein or it will be turned into sugar.' This is not a conclusion drawn often by anyone who understands nutrition.

Only when being in a state of ketosis is essential would you worry about how 'high' someone's protein was. Gluconeogenesis can bring someone out of a state of ketosis by converting protein into glucose. A lot of keto practitioners will monitor not only their carbohydrates but their protein too for this reason.

2. 'The body can only absorb 30g of protein in one sitting.'

This quite simply isn't true. The body can – and will – absorb more than 30g of protein in a sitting. The above quote is from a study in which **between 30g and 80g of protein was consumed and there was no benefit to the muscle protein synthesis** (MPS). However, there are plenty of roles for amino acids (protein) outside of MPS, let alone the process of gluconeogenesis, which, I know, sounds like a character from *The Matrix*. Amino acids help regulate immune function, nitrogen balance and even mineral absorption. You may be thinking about buying them in their branched chain supplemental forms, but I'd advise just aiming to hit the goals from protein sources.

Are our organs at risk from a high protein diet? Well, according to research: 'In male subjects with several years of experience with resistance training, chronic consumption of a diet high in protein had no harmful effects on any measures of health. **Furthermore, there was no change in body weight, fat mass, or lean body mass despite eating more total calories and protein.**' (See References, p.286.)

So that dispels the notion of consuming *too much protein being 'bad for us'*. As far as 'over-reaching' goes, we just need to consider that if we keep our calories the same and push protein up, fats and carbohydrates will have to come down to accommodate. Here's a simple way to look at it. The best diet for muscle growth is:

> When you're lean, train hard, consume 2–3g protein per kg and eat as much as you can without getting fat. If you start getting fat, dial it back a bit. In other words, reduce your calorie intake.

This is an intentionally reductive summation of gaining muscle without gaining fat, to show how simple the principle should be.

Carbohydrates are essential for optimal recovery in the context of refuelling our muscles and fuelling workouts, but in certain circumstances (albeit rarely), the body can convert protein into carbohydrates. However, that aside, the repercussions of being 30g over your protein target vs 30g under are **always going to favour being over the protein target in question**.

To conclude: overtraining is unlikely; however, over-reaching is very common. Listen to your body and ensure you're not forcing sessions. Better to take time off than to force it; better to go back to training later after an injury than earlier; and always better to overshoot your protein than under-consume it. Voila.

The bro split

What I call the 'bro split' is the overly popular and, unfortunately, widely accepted method of separating training into certain body parts and allocating an entire day to them, like this:

- ▸ Arms Day
- ▸ Back Day
- ▸ Legs Day
- ▸ Chest Day
- ▸ Shoulders Day

Embarrassingly, I'll admit that in my former professional corporate life I'd keep five bits of paper with these headings on them in a little pot and get Lynn, who sat opposite me, to pick what I was going to train that day. (You can see how dull my work life was – the randomness of this brought me a little excitement for my lunch break.)

This system has conveniently gained popularity by fitting into the work week for the gym bro (formerly me) who wants to lift and get so large and swollen he'd be likely to call himself 'Lord Swoledermort'. One of the patterns you'll start to realize in this part of the book is that much of the context has derived from anecdotal belief and not from the actual science. You could say largely from the beliefs of a younger, more naive version of … me.

The 'bro split' does have a place for some very experienced body-builders. Imagine that a gym session tailored towards muscle growth can last 45–80 minutes – that could easily be the right amount of time for a very experienced gym 'bro' to get enough stimulus on his, let's say, 'Arms Day' for growth. The main issue is that Linda from Norwich is now having a Shoulders Day set in her training regime, and I want to bring the science to light a bit here to stop people from daft programming or, even worse, dull programming, which is going to get Linda back to daft home workouts faster than you can shake a sheep's tail.

Over the years I have had to remind many personal trainers that they are not their clients. All too often, I look around and I see the trainer getting their client to do their own workout, just slightly modified for the person paying them. Now, you should realize that a lot of PTs are also bodybuilders, many of whom practise a lot of pseudoscience. And another thing to remember is that you can get strong with bad form and you can get in good shape with poor practices. I mean, you could literally only eat chicken and broccoli and only do a bro split and, in enough time, I'm sure you'd look great – it's just not necessary, that's my biggest concern.

Training a body part in a bro fashion is not BAD, it's just not quite getting your 'bang for your buck', nor is it the optimal way of doing things for what I perceive to be the reader of this book. Another thing to take into account is that unfortunately, muscle physiology does not play by the rules of the seven-day week. For this reason, training a body part – say, legs once a week – is not damaging; it's just not allowing the person to reach their full potential. This is my opinion, of course, so let me tell you a James Smith story.

I'm lying back in the dentist's chair in Sydney. My dentist flashes me the background on his phone in a discussion about training. I notice the bloke is in amazing condition. I think to myself, Holy shit – my dentist is in better shape than I am. When he takes his tools out my mouth, I compliment him on his 'rig', as I'd call it. He says, 'Oh, that's not me – that's, in fact, the body I want.' I proceed to let him know why he should not have that there, comparison being the thief of joy and all that. I ask him about his current split, and lo and behold, it's the omni-present 'bro split'. My brain neurons fire and my finest skill comes to light as I decide to create a flossing analogy.

So I say to my dentist: hypothetically, every minute of flossing repre-sents a set completed of an exercise on a body part. So I floss for twenty-one minutes, representing twenty-one sets of an exercise, let's say legs, for instance. Now, twenty-one sets of legs is a fairly normal amount for a 45–80-minute 'bro legs' session. It may be four to five sets of squats, four to five sets of deadlifts or Romanian variants. It could be four sets of standing calves, four sets of seated calves and some leg extensions or glutes work to finish. You could walk out of the gym like John Wayne and tweet about how much of a hero you are*

Twenty-one minutes of flossing per week is enough to arouse any dentist. Until, that is, I say that I intend to floss the full twenty-one minutes on just one day a week. I then propose to my dentist the idea of flossing instead the same amount of time overall, but three times a week for seven minutes a go. It's the same amount of flossing – all I'd do is increase the frequency, and we'd see a superior return on oral hygiene, right?

Now, oral hygiene and muscle growth are not identical, but you get the idea. Rather than doing an hour of legs, where fatigue can kick in very soon (especially in the relatively untrained), it's a better idea to allocate smaller periods of time to accomplish the stimulus we would like. I personally wouldn't advocate anyone do a bro split unless they are very experienced or they're on anabolic steroids (which I also do not recommend).

* It's worth noting DOMS (delayed onset muscle soreness) usually occurs two days after training but lasts no longer than four days typically. This is an indicator of the full cycle of stimulus to recovery. Muscle soreness is inflammation, keep that in mind for the pub quiz in case it ever comes up, but it's not a sliding scale where more DOMS = better results.

Looking at the science, it does actually slightly contradict my theory: 'Under volume-equated conditions, Resistance Training frequency does not seem to have a pronounced effect of gains in muscle mass.' (See References, p.286.)

However, I still have a reason for advocating a more frequent split, which isn't discussed in the above conclusion. I feel that in untrained and even intermediate trainees, greater training frequency can allow not only **a greater volume of training each week**, but an improved intensity, without being undone by fatigue, **not to mention the importance of enjoyment when training for the untrained and intermediates to encourage adherence and sustainability** i.e. people enjoying their workouts.

To conclude, although matching volume (the number of sets performed in a week) is the key underlying factor in muscle growth, it's worth noting that increasing the frequency of sessions (how many times a body part is trained) may not, on its own, elicit more muscle growth. However, the effects of a more sensible split and a higher intensity could – and usually do – lead to increased volume of training before fatigue sets in. I think it's also very important for us to realize that not everyone either wants to or enjoys training an entire body part for the duration of a session, even if they're physically able to. If someone's first session with a PT consists of training a body part for an hour to extreme fatigue, I very much think that could reduce the chances of that person coming back.

So let's say Leg-Day Lewis has just welcomed Linda into the gym for her Shoulders Day. Linda is relatively untrained, and ten minutes or even four to five sets is more than enough for muscle growth to occur in her shoulders. Now, my problem is not with people training, especially not weight training. I just have an issue with the fact that it could be done better without much having to change for the person in question. Let's say Linda comes to me and asks on the spot what I would get her to do instead. I could prescribe her a training split that looks a little like this:

Monday (20–30 minutes)
4x sets squats
3x sets leg extensions
(then train another area of choice)

Wednesday (20–30 minutes)
4x sets barbell hip thrusts
3x sets Romanian deadlifts
(then train another area of choice)

Friday (20–30 minutes)
3x Bulgarian split squats
2x lying hamstring curls
2x seated abductions
(then train another area of choice)

Linda would see the same volume (twenty-one sets), but with a more even split. This means more frequent bouts of stimulation and recovery. Not only that, but her intensity can remain higher during a shorter period of work. Now, I've assumed Linda's goals here, but with only perhaps twenty minutes taken up, it means she can train other body parts on the same day. Push movements include bench press, shoulder press and dips.* Pull movements are rows, upright rows and pulldowns.

* For video tutorials on these movements and more, visit www.jamessmithacademy.com.

She now can train legs (above) for twenty minutes three times a week and do the same with push movements (chest and triceps) and pull movements (back and biceps).

Poor Linda nearly dropped a week's wages to go with Lewis to train shoulders for an hour. Instead she could have done seven very difficult sets of legs, seven very difficult sets of push and seven very difficult sets of pull. It would take the same time as the twenty-one sets of shoulders that Lewis had planned.

Fat burners

The large majority of supplements serve no tangible purpose, as I mentioned in Part 1, and you'll see again in this chapter, but one thing I want to call out is this notion of supplementing 'fat burners'. In almost all cases, these are just stimulants.

In the metabolic adaptation and adaptive thermogenesis section (aka starvation mode – see p.182), we saw a decrease in energy output when dieting, and this only becomes more severe the leaner someone becomes. For this reason, to keep their non-resting energy expenditure as high as possible (NREE), I'd give them stimulants to keep them up and moving, and I could even see an increase in the gym duration, intensity and someone's step count when stimulated vs not stimulated. Even refraining from a nap could mean a higher energy output.

According to research: 'Based on the available literature, caffeine and green tea have data to back up its fat metabolism-enhancing properties. For many other supplements, although some show some promise, evidence is lacking. The list of supplements is industry-driven and is likely to grow at a rate that is not matched by a similar increase in scientific underpinning.' (See References, p.287.) The main ingredient in many 'fat burners' is caffeine. Now, there's not a huge amount of solid evidence correlating caffeine to fat loss; however, as I'm sure you can imagine, someone who feels energized will probably burn more calories than someone who is not. It's still important to note, though, that not everyone responds to caffeine, and also that we can't draw a conclusion on its efficacy without knowing how many calories a person has consumed vs the next person, not to mention their genetic differences – it's a minefield. 'The major findings from this study indicate that ingestion of a thermogenic fat-loss supplement containing approximately 200mg of caffeine, green tea extract and other ingredients can significantly increase RMR (resting metabolic rate) over a three-hour time period in healthy males. These elevations came with no adverse effects relative to resting heart rate and only slight increases in blood pressure values. Although the thermogenic fat-loss supplement resulted in an elevation in RMR, **at this time we are not able to conclude whether this can lead to actual fat loss over time in this group**.' (See References, p.287.)

So we can't just say caffeine = fat loss.

Instead, we can say that in some people it can help with the number of calories burned at rest. I feel the best place to draw a conclusion would be to identify caffeine's role in improving sports performance *and therefore our own performance*: 'Caffeine can be used effectively as an ergogenic* aid when taken in moderate doses, such as during sports when a small increase in endurance performance can lead to significant differences in placements as athletes are often separated by small margins.' (See References, p.287.)

I don't want to delve too far into the illegal substances because that would simultaneously raise awareness of them, but it's worth knowing what is often used in the fitness industry.

The most common 'fat burner' I see used is Clenbuterol. It's an asthma drug which is commonly used as a stimulant; it slightly raises your metabolic rate and your temperature (thermogenesis), which means you'll burn more calories at rest. There are some other more complex mechanisms, which mean you'd be in a good position for

* Ergogenic: an ergogenic aid can be broadly defined as a technique or substance used for the purpose of enhancing performance. Ergogenic aids have been classified as nutritional, pharmacologic, physiologic or psychologic and range from use of accepted techniques such as carbohydrate loading to illegal and unsafe approaches such as anabolic-androgenic steroid use.

losing body fat. Now, although this seems like a fantastic drug to take, it comes with a plethora of potential dangers to cardiac health and other side effects that aren't too nice, ranging from palpitations, tremors, anxiety and severe cramps – which usually strike when trying to do something simple like use a pen or even when you try to fall asleep at night. So again, from experience: stay sensible, people.

To conclude, there are no compounds or supplements that 'burn fat' as such, but there are substances that can increase your activity, decrease your responses to caloric restriction (adaptive thermogenesis) and substances that are abused to elicit faster fat loss, albeit potentially to the detriment of overall health.

Supplements

When looking at supplementing our diets, it's important to note that the large majority of supplements on offer do from very little to fuck all to benefit us in the long run. As I explained in the sleep section (see p.90), you're better off going to bed earlier than spending hundreds of pounds on supplements, in my personal opinion.

The only two supplements I will exclude from that statement are whey protein and creatine.

Whey protein

'It's filtered fucking milk, mate,' you'll hear me say across social-media videos. Whey protein is created in the process of cheese-making, would you believe? After the curd is strained, the remaining liquid is whey. And here's what you need to know about whey protein:

- ▸ Some people who are dairy 'intolerant' are, in fact, just in a pickle because they do not produce enough or any of an enzyme called lactase, which is needed to break down lactose (a sugar present in milk). If this applies to you, it does not mean you have to avoid whey; instead try whey isolate – I've found that unflavoured versions of this are the easiest to supplement for those who are 'lactose intolerant' to avoid any stomach upset.
- ▸ Whey protein is fast absorbed and has what is known as a great 'amino acid' profile. It's a good source of protein (when choosing foods for protein there are subtle differences, but it's not worth getting bogged down in).

- Whey protein doesn't need to be cooked and can be kept at room temperature – not only that, but it's much more socially acceptable to shake in a shaker while walking around the office at 4 p.m. than shaking a chicken breast in front of onlooking colleagues.

To conclude, **whey protein is more of a superfood than a supplement**. We don't see many people proclaim that cheese is a supplement, so let's begin a movement of seeing it as a powdered, convenient, well-priced food *that anyone striving for optimal composition would have in their diet.*

The main difference between brands in my experience is in how they are marketed by supplement companies, but the truth is many of them are very similar. Annoyingly, most people rate them on taste, and I don't recall many fitness enthusiasts taking them to the lab for testing on quality before advising you on what's the best protein for you.

Creatine

I get asked about creatine daily. Creatine is one of the most popular and widely researched supplement. The majority of studies have focused on the effects of creatine monohydrate on performance and health; however, many other forms of creatine exist and are commercially available in the sports nutrition/supplement market. Regardless of the form, supplementation with creatine has regularly shown to increase strength, fat-free mass and muscle shape and structure.

Creatine is produced endogenously (internally) at an amount of about 1g a day. Synthesis (production) of creatine predominantly occurs in the liver, kidneys and, to a lesser extent, in the pancreas. The remainder of the creatine available to the body is obtained through the diet at about 1g a day for an omnivorous diet. Ninety-five per cent of the body's creatine distribution is found in the skeletal muscle. As creatine is mainly present in the diet in meats, vegetarians and vegans typically have lower resting creatine concentrations.

Research reviews indicate that creatine supplementation has a positive impact on:

- amplifying the effects of resistance training for enhancing strength and muscle growth
- improving the quality and benefits of high-intensity intermittent speed training
- improving aerobic endurance performance
- strength, power, fat-free mass, daily living performance and neurological function in young and older people (See References, p.287.)

The benefits of creatine to those suffering from sleep deprivation are now emerging as well: 'Following 24-hour sleep deprivation, creatine supplementation had a positive effect on mood state and tasks that place a heavy stress on the brain.' (See References, p.287.)

So as you can see, for those wishing to get the most out of their performance, **creatine is an addition that actually is effective in providing a range of benefits outside physical performance**. Not only that, but it is well priced too.

Are there any dangers in supplementing with creatine?

There's a lot of literature about creatine use in adolescent athletes suggesting that it appears to be well tolerated with **no reported adverse effects**. (See References, p.287.) We cannot dismiss the now twenty-five plus years of research that continues to highlight that creatine use in a multitude of populations **is safe and effective**.

So, as you can see, creatine is effective and safe. I have it daily when possible; usually just put it in with my whey protein shake. For some, it can cause a stomach ache, and there's no way to find out if that is you until you supplement it. If that's the case, I'm unaware of any way around that at this moment.

What do you need to know about creatine supplementation?

- Monohydrate is the only version you'll need
- Creatine can require a loading phase to 'saturate' stores. However, typically, I just start the recommended dose daily and set a reminder on my phone to take it every day
- Creatine can benefit as a placebo in the onset, but remember if a placebo works, it works

Non-essential supplementation

I've stressed many times before that usually the people I know who are in the best shape supplement the least and those who are in not such great shape tend to supplement the most.

I am going to mention some of the mainstream supplements on p.212, and I'll attach what the science says (probably to the chagrin of the big supplement companies). The most annoying thing is how often people say to me, **'But James – can you show me how it doesn't work?'** This is the wrong question to be asking. Instead, we should be challenging the efficacy of the supplement in the first place! Not only that, but supplements that yield such acute changes in whatever way they claim need to be disregarded and instead priority shunted on to those things that really do create tangible and noticeable changes, like sleep and nutrition.

Here's a reminder of our 'good life' pyramids:

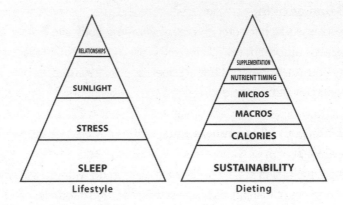

Lifestyle   Dieting

Branched Chain Amino Acids – BCAAs

I must admit, as a PT I was guilty of supplementing these for a long time. In my head, I always have the argument that 'if a placebo works, it works'. However, these supplements are not cheap, and as if protein in itself didn't cost the average fitness person an arm and a leg, I don't think anyone deserves the 'stupid tax' of paying for BCAAs on top.

Amino acids form protein, the 'building blocks', so to speak. So I thought that having these in circulation would only benefit me and 'protect' my muscle when unfed, dieting or training.

Turns out there's no need for these supplements at all, according to the science, keeping in mind we have two hours' training's worth of muscle glycogen most of the time, plus, if we are hitting our protein targets (1.5–2.5g per kg) there should be sufficient amino acids in circulation. There's emerging data surrounding BCAAs helping with DOMS (muscle soreness), but I don't think they warrant necessity among anyone I have trained in the past or anyone I am likely to train in the future.

The complex part:

Protein is required for growth and repair of the body and tissues. The amount is usually chosen relative to the size of the person – that's why I have put 'per kilogram' throughout this book. If you're carrying a fair bit of timber (fat), it's a good idea to choose an amount of protein that is relatively close to your lean mass (without fat). So if you're 100kg and have a feeling you're carrying around 20kg of fat – your lean body mass (the amount of mass without fat on it) would be 80kg.

Now, the sliding scale (1.5–2.5g) has more to do with your goal and environment of training. If you're someone getting into fitness and it's your first time calculating your protein goal, I recommend the lower end of 1.5g per kg (use my calculator on www.jamessmithacademy. com/calculator). To most of the fitness industry, this is considered fairly low; however, for someone new to this way of eating, I think it's the perfect amount to maximize the benefits of higher protein without flipping someone's diet and way of eating upside down.

If you're dieting in a big deficit or looking to maximize muscle growth, then it's worth aiming for the higher ranges – up to 2.5g per kg. I weigh about 91kg without much fat, so that's 227.5g of protein a day.

The important thing here is that weight is not the weight of the protein source itself. For instance, a chicken breast may weigh 100g and only have 10–20g of protein in it. To give you a visual idea of 227.5g of protein – it's give or take ten scoops of whey protein, which is circa 25g a scoop. That's not to say you should drink ten shakes a day; it's just to give you an idea of how much that is for me.

Linda from Norwich is looking to lose 10kg. She's currently weighing 79kg. Let's decide she's 69kg lean and she's relatively new to dieting. So we take 69kg x 1.5g = 103.5g protein per day. That could be a scoop of whey with a yoghurt for breakfast (40g) followed by a salmon salad at lunch (25g), some chocolate rice cakes mid-afternoon before exercising (0g), a shake post-workout (25g), then for dinner she'd only require 20g, which could easily fit into any traditional dish she's cooking with her family or friends.*

What does the scientific literature say?

'There is a paucity of evidence supporting a beneficial effect for BCAA supplementation in promoting increases in muscle protein synthesis or lean mass.' (See References, p.287.)

I had to google that one. Some of the evidence out there when examined is incorrect. Often companies will 'sponsor' a study to go ahead and the findings usually conveniently come back with the best interest of the sponsor.

To conclude. There's no real reason or benefit for anyone to supplement BCAAs in a calorie deficit or even in a state of looking to build muscle. **Focus should be on total protein intake from food.** It's a shame because most mainstream training plans that we see recommend BCAA supplementation with a 'discount code'. Unfortunately, these are, in fact, commission codes for the person who has written the plan. Same goes for leucine, which we will look at next.

Leucine

Leucine is an amino acid very popular in mainstream training programmes. It has the capacity to stimulate something called 'muscle protein synthesis' – a form of muscle-building machinery, let's say. Leucine tends to be found in lower amounts in foods that form vegan

* For food and recipe ideas, calorie calculator and a breakdown of how to use tracking software, go to www.jamessmithacademy.com.

and vegetarian diets, so for people following those diets I would recommend either supplementing it (only if striving for optimal muscle growth) with each feeding, or increasing protein amounts at each meal in order to hit the amount of leucine required for MPS.

'Vegan athletes, however, appear to consume less protein than their omnivorous and vegetarian counterparts. The optimisation of protein intakes for vegan athletes requires that attention is paid to the quantity and quality of protein consumed. Plant-based protein sources are often incomplete, missing important essential amino acids, and typically contain less Branched Chain Amino Acids (BCAA) than their animal-based equivalents. Leucine appears to be a primary trigger of MPS, and plays an important role in promoting recovery and adaptation from exercise.' (See References, p.287.)

To conclude, leucine is something to consider if you're serious about gaining muscle at the same time as being vegetarian/vegan. If not, *save your money*.

The others

L-carnitine, apple cider vinegar and glutamine are other high-street products that promise the world. I'd love to tell you they do fuck all, but the science can sometimes show acute benefits with use which quickly discontinues afterwards. So rather than slander their efficacy, I think it's best for us to realize that there is no point parting with our money for these supplements when we could yield a superior response from being smart with our training, resting appropriately, splitting training in the right manner and getting the adequate amount of sleep that we need, not to mention prioritizing high-quality nutrition. Basically, putting into practice what you have learned so far in this book.

Skinny teas, coffees and 'weight-loss shots'

Unfortunately, we're living in a world where people are more desperate than ever to look a certain way – the same as their idols on social media. Because of this, they're more likely to succumb to social-media marketing. You start to realize it may not be so difficult to lure young teenage girls or a new mother struggling with her weight to buy a brightly coloured pink 'weight-loss shot' that you mix with water, having seen it advertised across social media, endorsed by a Z-list celebrity, targeting someone's insecurities while simultaneously increasing them. That, paired with screen times upwards of five hours a day on smartphones, and it's easy to see how people are lured into buying these fat-loss products that promise the world and often deliver nothing in return.

'Skinny' branded coffee is just decaffeinated coffee. That's it. Look at the back of the packaging and that's the ingredients. It's advised to drink before bed. If I told my mum I was going to drink decaf coffee before bed in a bid to lose weight, she'd call me daft. Yet a load of the nation are paying an arm and a leg for some overpriced decaf and having it before bed – surely, after the sleep part of the book (see p.90) you know that's counterintuitive, right?

Weight-loss shots. Whenever I see them a bit of me dies inside. The main ingredient is a 'natural appetite suppressant' known as gluco-mannan. So what does the science say?

'Glucomannan supplements were well tolerated but **did not promote weight loss in overweight and moderately obese individuals** consuming self-selected diets and maintaining usual physical activity patterns. (…) Given the growing epidemic of obesity, additional studies to assess the safety and efficacy of this widely used alternative weight loss approach are needed.' (See References, p.287.)

In time I'd like to see legislation where any new product to the market must first prove its efficacy before finding its way onto shelves or on the news feeds of Instagram Z-list celebrities trying to make a few quid.

Artificial sweeteners

These have been a subject of debate for quite some time. In the UK we for some reason call Coca-Cola the 'full-fat' version when we are describing any variant that isn't 'diet'.

'Oh, sweeteners are bad for you; you're actually best off drinking the full-fat version.' I have been guilty of saying this at least a handful of times when I used to do my 'research' from Google and articles from Dr Mercola, back in the day, stating that sweeteners caused dementia, heart disease and stroke.

However, if I managed to keep my head out of other people's opinions, I would conclude that surely a beverage without calories vs one with them would be the better choice?

Artificial sweeteners provide greater food choices to people looking to cut down calories and improve the palatability of food. However, many of their purported beneficial effects remain invalidated in large-scale clinical studies. I feel this is due to the fact that someone who has no idea what energy balance or calorie deficit is, nor do they understand many factors in fat loss, will probably drink a Diet Coke. Not only that but, of course, someone overweight or obese will also pick a Diet Coke, due to external societal pressures in a shop, restaurant, etc.

But association is not causation, remember? For that reason, just because many obese people drink Diet Coke and don't successfully lose fat by doing so, it doesn't mean it's ineffective when implemented correctly as part of a calorie-controlled regimen.

What does the science say? Aspartame is the most common and prevalent sweetener spoken about in mainstream media and, contrary to popular belief, it doesn't affect your appetite, glucose or insulin levels and can, therefore, save you lots of calories in your diet, making subtle swaps and changes resulting in relatively easy weight loss.

Aspartame is a form of artificial sweetener, technically labelled as food additive E951, which is one of the feared E numbers. This E-number talk crops up with many 'clean-eating' gurus as though they're something terrible and bad – like, 'Oh my God, I wouldn't eat that.' I've even heard people try to label E numbers as the reason why kids can't concentrate at school, as well as a host of other things. **But there are over a thousand other E numbers and hundreds of them are artificial. The E number is actually a symbol of safety and it means the EU have classified it safe for human consumption.**

Menno Henselmans – a highly regarded nutrition researcher – created a fantastic infographic showing that if you consume one can of diet soda with 125mg of aspartame in it, the aspartame will break down into three substances very quickly:

10 per cent of it will be broken down into methanol.
Sounds scary, but a glass of tomato juice contains six times as much.

40 per cent is broken down into aspartic acid.
Sounds frightening, but one egg contains thirty-four times as much.

50 per cent of it is broken down into phenylalanine.
Unpronounceable and scary, yet 100g of beef contains sixteen to
thirty-two times as much.*

The most recent research shows that aspartame is broken down so fast
it can't have a negative impact on the gut. (See References, p.287.) Also,
the most recent review paper confirms that aspartame poses no harm
to health. (See References, p.287.)

To conclude, artificial sweeteners should not be demonized outright.
When implemented correctly they can play a very positive role in reducing calories. It's better to consume diet drinks than continue to consume
vast amounts of calories through 'full fat' (i.e. full sugar) soda drinks. It's
better to have aspartame in your system for a short period than increase
your risk of cardiovascular disease and other obesity-related illnesses
through over-consumption of calories on a chronic basis.

Even with what the FDA concludes is a safe amount of aspartame, I
calculated I could consume dozens of cans of Diet Coke a day with no
problems. Of course, water is king, but if you're on a calorie-controlled
diet, then reach for the diet soda before any 'full fat' option.

* Menno Henselmans @menno.henselmans

Weight regain

Head onto Twitter and search #antidiet and it won't take long to find someone in high-waisted leggings proclaiming: 'Diets don't work!' They'll talk about the contestants on *The Biggest Loser* and waffle on about weight regain or even the theory of 'set point', whereby our weight is controlled by a biological set point determined by our DNA. However, this theory is more of a control for weight loss rather than weight gain – to bring the person **back up** to their 'set point' from a period of dieting.

Set-point theory

There have been an abundance of studies looking into this over the years, even assessing people on starvation diets of 50 per cent of their calories for twenty-four weeks – for example, the Minnesota Starvation Experiment.

In the Minnesota Starvation Experiment, conducted between 1944 and 1945, the subjects lost 66 per cent of their fat mass in response to twenty-four weeks of semi-starvation (i.e. at 50 per cent reduced energy intake), but ad libitum refeeding resulted in a regain of fat mass reaching 145 per cent of their pre-starvation values (i.e. there was an overshooting of fat mass, known as the catch-up fat phenomenon). Thus, the fluctuation in body weight that results from under- and overfeeding requires a considerable change in the hypothetical set point, at least after starvation, refeeding and overeating. (See References, p.287.)

I can't help but feel that the large majority of people use their set point as a scapegoat for their lack of progress in sustainable fat loss or composition. People are very quick to point the finger at their genetics, but it's nearly impossible to determine if that holds true due to the rapidly changing environments that we're exposed to. Generation by generation, environment and socioeconomics, not to mention the culture of eating, change incredibly fast.

For instance, within one generation from my parents to me, we now have Deliveroo, Uber, electric bikes on every corner and smartphones that can even dim the lights in my front room without my having to stand up. It's all too easy to blame our genetics or a theoretical 'set point' for how much fat we have gained and accrued over the past few months and years, but we need to look elsewhere too.

And the fundamental elements of our environment that impact on our energy-balance equation carry across from species to species: **a growing level of canine obesity is associated with snack eating and low socioeconomic state**, therefore suggesting that the overweight issue is not just a human problem, nor a 'genetics' problem, but more down to the environment a given species exists within.

Regaining weight 'with interest'

'Ninety-five per cent of everyone who loses weight regains it back, with interest.' I can't stand this type of talk. Who does it benefit? Even if it was true, it's not something we should remind people of. We could classify it in the category of, 'Good morning. Just thought I'd remind you that you're going to die. Have a good day!' Or, 'Do you know what you could have bought with all the money you paid to the taxman this year?' Or, 'Good night. Oh, just to remind you that statistically you hugely underestimate the chances of your dying from a terminal condition before you're sixty.'

Thanks, mate. Great chat. I'm pretty sure this originated from an ancient study and it's still mainstream talk to this day. Now, before I get into a meta-analysis of US studies, I want to make two things clear:

- ▸ A meta-analysis is a procedure for combining data from multiple studies
- ▸ Most methods of losing fat are pretty shite

The majority of weight-loss studies are *not* done in health-seeking, fit, young people who want to be a part of an experiment for shits and giggles. Usually, they tend to use people who are very eager to lose fat and most probably to avoid health issues soon likely to arise. This means that they can stick to a very restrictive diet with the pressure of their health on the line. **But their habits aren't always addressed or changed in the way they need to be.** Say that person is 50kg overweight before they do the study, they lose a large proportion of that weight, but all they have done is barely eat for several weeks/months. What about their work, their gym routine, their family or work commitments – what about all the causes that got them to be 50kg overweight in the first place? **If those roots of the cause are not addressed it's only likely they'll regain weight.**

In the Vietnam War, at least one in five US soldiers – whether to deal with the stress of the war or hedonistic tendencies – took heroin and marijuana. Heroin is an incredibly addictive drug, and there were great concerns over the number of soldiers who would come home addicted and therefore needing rehab. Yet when returning to the USA, most of the men who had used it in Vietnam used it very rarely or not at all.

This is to do with the environment the participant is in at the time. *The Biggest Loser* contestants were taken into an alien environment where they trained hard and dieted, then thrown back into the lives they came from. Habits and environment are closely linked together and it's why people can dramatically change their lifestyle, the way they dress and the shape they're in when relocating, whether it is for a job or a loved one.

So we need also to be mindful of people being dieted down and then thrown back into their old lifestyle, where they are surrounded by the people, cues, shops and habits that caused them to be a part of a trial in the first place.

What does the science say?

A meta-analysis of twenty-nine reports of long-term weight-loss maintenance indicated that four or five years after a structured weight-loss programme weight loss was maintained. (See References, p.288.)

So as we can see from this meta-analysis, the weight regain statistic of '95 per cent of diets fail' is quite simply not true. Not only that, but it is irresponsible to claim this in the first place. How can anyone truly know what percentage of dieters regain weight?

To conclude, even with a large proportion of methods for sustainable fat loss being awful, the notion of weight regain is not backed by the scientific experiments and the 'set-point' theory is influenced by environment and socioeconomic status more than our genetics or DNA. It's certainly not another barrier to put between you and your next period of dieting.

Cheat meals

The way we communicate with ourselves is more important than we may think, and even how we label certain situations is important. I am guilty for having glorified the 'cheat meal' back in the day as a gym bro, BCAA enthusiast and part-time meathead, but now I've done a 180 turnaround and I don't like the terminology one bit. I'll explain why.

When drilling down into the concept of the 'cheat meal', I often use the analogy of the thousands of people who go to Ibiza each year on holiday. They go to well-known beach clubs and buy bottles of champagne for thousands of pounds. Now, some people can afford to waste such money on ridiculous mark-ups. For the large majority it's something they save all year for, to blow on one day. This is any person's prerogative and I'm not saying they can't do it. I'm just saying *there is a more sensible approach.*

A cheat meal is when someone takes a break from dieting and has a meal they deem as a 'cheat' from their diet – these can range from hundreds to potentially thousands of calories per sitting, which are usually 'discounted' by the dieter because they are within the context of the 'cheat meal'. But I think there are some important things to note.

You decide to have a 'cheat meal'; you order a large pepperoni pizza from Domino's, which is 3,040 calories, and the garlic bread, which is 328 calories. But you're a smart cookie and have a Diet Coke, as you're currently reading my book.

That's 3,368 calories. Let's call it 3,400. Cool, your prerogative. Now a few things from me:

- ▶ Just call it what it is, a fucking calorie-dense meal. Calling it a 'cheat' doesn't do anything productive; it doesn't reduce the calories or increase the thermic effect of food. You could call your pizza Trisha or bloody Chuck Norris, but the fact of the matter is that labelling it as a cheat reinforces the thinking that you're having to cheat from a protocol. Cheating in a relationship is bad and usually means the relationship isn't working – in the same way, you could infer that you're breaking a diet that isn't working.
- ▶ As well as nailing that amount of calories in a sitting (never mind other food in that day), I very much doubt you're going

to be feeling like moving too much after that pizza. So your TDEE would be negatively influenced in a lot of ways. Instead, what about enjoying another 485 calories EACH DAY during the week?

This could not only fuel workouts and aid in recovery from training, but be added to evening meals to accommodate cooking alongside family and friends or social occasions. To put into perspective the 485 calories that you could have each day:

- two cinnamon and raisin bagels
- five and a half chocolate-covered rice cakes
- one McDonald's chicken ranch wrap
- three quarters of a bag of Percy Pigs (UK sweets)
- one and a half tubs of Halo Top ice cream

Now, I've listed hedonic, pleasurable foods and you could opt for something healthier, but the point I want to make clear is that you need to ask yourself this: 'Would consuming these foods more frequently diminish my want for a binge at the weekend?'

Because that's what a 'cheat meal' is: it's a justified binge, so that any fitness professional can remove guilt by snapping a picture, sitting next to it and posting #cheatmeal. Also, I feel with my clients that if I wish to drop someone's calories – whether for faster fat loss, a plateau from adaptive thermogenesis or their sheer frustration from slow progress – I can dial back the daily food: two fewer rice cakes, one fewer bagel, etc., rather than have the other conversation of eradicating an entire cheat meal that could be their much-needed psychological break from dieting. Otherwise, it's: 'Ah, Simon, mate – as part of creating a larger deficit, I need you to only eat three quarters of that pizza!' Who in their right mind is going to walk away from a pizza with a couple of slices left? Not me; not anyone sane, anyway.

So to conclude, call it what it is: a calorie-dense meal. Instead of demonizing it as a cheat, just deal with it and the repercussions. You log and you learn; next time you might go for a thin crust or even a burger and chips instead and save 1,000 calories. Best of all, why not include foods that previously have made you feel bad or 'guilty'? I'll let you in on a case study with one of my face-to-face clients, Lauren.

FAT LOSS WITH REESE'S PIECES?

Lauren came to me in what I deemed already great shape. She wanted to lose a bit of fat and felt a bit clueless around the gym, using bits of equipment. So I took Lauren on and we trained for forty-five minutes, three times a week. I set Lauren's calories at 1,700 each day, which she thought seemed high, but seeing as she was already in good shape, I told her not to be daft. She also told me she'd been on 1,200 calories per day in the past and wasn't seeing any change. I set her protein goal at 120g minimum a day and obviously told her to choose the best quality foods possible.

She messaged me about three days in, saying: 'James, if I have 250 calories left and I've hit my protein target can I eat what I like?' I said for sure. She told me her vice was Reese's Pieces – a type of peanut butter chocolate treat. I said to go for it. She couldn't believe that she could eat them. I saw her at the tail end of the week and she was nervous, having eaten them most days, but I asked her to trust the process.

Three to four weeks in, her friends even made remarks on her physique and how much it was improving. She couldn't believe it either. This is where I thought I'd defied the law of thermodynamics because I had a client who'd eaten more food and lost more fat. I wasn't sure how on earth I was doing it either. About two weeks after that, Lauren told me that for the first time ever she'd actually started tracking weekends while training with me. 'James, when I was on 1,200 calories, by the time the weekend came around I ate everything, I'd binge on Reese's Pieces and not start logging until Monday again.' I asked her what happened now. She told me that because she eats just a few of them each day during the week, she's more than happy to only have a small amount or even leave them out for a glass of wine with friends at the weekend. For once she wasn't letting her weekend 'all-or-nothing' approach get in the way or throw her off course. Eating more during her week meant eating more sensibly at the weekends and not only *feeling* in control, but *being* in control.

So once again. if you want a calorie-dense meal, cool. But there are more sensible approaches that you may stick to better. Weekends are where diets can be won or lost; if you want to indulge, make it fit rather than making it a 'cheat'.

Fasted cardio

I was once a believer in fasted cardio being the ultimate method of burning fat. It makes sense, right? Unfed, fat to be used as a fuel source. Burn as much of it off as possible and then get on with your day of 'eating clean', right?

So first we have the question: 'Does eating inhibit our ability to burn fat?'

Well, here's one of my Instagram posts on the topic.

Firstly, let's distinguish two things:

Fat oxidation – fat being converted into energy.
Fat loss – the amount (or mass) of fat decreasing.

When we eat there is a rise in insulin, the hormone that helps maintain blood-sugar levels. It rises the most when we consume carbohydrates, although we produce it all the time in smaller amounts.

When insulin rises (fed state) fat oxidation stops, but this does not mean fat loss can't be achieved.

Similarly, imagine when you charge your iPhone and plug it in (feeding). There is no requirement for the phone to use its battery with a source of mains electricity coming into it.

Whether that iPhone has battery at the end of the day is dependent on amount of charge IN vs amount of phone use OUT.

Whether fat oxidation is high or low at time of training will not impact fat loss more or less positively, as that's governed by energy IN vs OUT.

You don't get an Uber surcharge rate of 1.4x just because you trained fasted. If you really want to nit-pick, you could argue that fed workouts lead to better performance and endurance.

So therefore, should calories and protein stay the same, the fed trainees could expend more calories, creating a larger deficit and superior fat loss (but not oxidation).

So on this I usually let people know that it's personal preference for the win here. If you want to eat, eat; if you don't, don't! There's nothing inherently wrong with training fasted. I just don't want people to believe it's superior because it's not. If someone wakes up starving and really wants to eat, I want them to know that eating is okay – it won't hinder their fat-loss efforts if they stick to the same amount of food they were going to eat anyway.

And what about the science?

Well, in 2014, Brad Schoenfeld and a few other highly regarded nutrition researchers did one of the first studies to determine whether being in a fasted state would be superior for fat loss vs fed.

They concluded that body composition changes associated with aerobic exercise in conjunction with a hypocaloric diet are similar, regardless of whether or not an individual is fasted prior to training, so those seeking to lose body fat can choose to train either before or after eating, based on preference. (See References, p.288.)

So to conclude, when we're seeking to make changes to our body fat, whether it is to increase or decrease that mass, we need to look at total volumes of calories in vs out and, of course, to remember the different thermic effects and satiety indexes of those foods. Eating a higher-protein diet, for instance, would have a far superior effect to benefit a proposed calorie deficit compared to a focus on training in a fasted state.

Low-carb diets and keto

Low-carbohydrate diets have been hugely popular for years now. Let's imagine our calories in the form of their macronutrient make-up. Now, this isn't me saying that you should walk around a supermarket like it's *The Matrix* and only see Carbs, Fats and Proteins – I want you to identify it as real food. But understanding where foods sit within these just makes your life of dieting simpler, easier and will improve the efficacy of whatever you implement.

So to create a calorie deficit, we need to reduce the amount of some macronutrients. Now, each macronutrient has a certain amount of calories or energy per gram, which isn't to say they are good or bad, just that some are denser than others.

Dietary fats contain 9 calories per gram.

You flip over an item of food to see that according to the label, it contains 20g fat. So you now know that it contains 180kcals of dietary fats – not good, not bad, just something to be aware of. I like logging foods in mainstream restaurants occasionally to see the content and to my surprise I see large inclusions of dietary fats – again, not to say a food is 'bad', I just want to know the make-up of what I order. For instance, Bang Bang Cauliflower at Wagamama, which is considered a starter, contains 474 calories – you saw previously what that equates to (five rice cakes, two bagels, etc. – see p.223). I check MyFitnessPal and see it has 32g of fat. I ask Siri what 32 x 9 is and I realize that 288 calories of the cauliflower is coming from fat. I decide to pick something more satiating. Again, not to demonize dietary fats, but they are the most dense when it comes to calories, and most likely to be in foods without us knowing.

NOTE ON DIETARY FATS

Whenever dieting anyone, I'd never want to drop their level of dietary fats below 20 per cent, as a ball park figure, of total make-up of calories.

It's important we don't go too low with fats as we need them for many biological processes, and if you remember from the sleep section of the book (see p.90), dropping them too low can negatively impact on your sex drive, among other issues. Links have also been suggested between very low-fat diets and metabolic syndrome.* (See References, p.288.)

It's easy to understand why dietary fats have been an easy target to slash in a bid to lose fat, due to their calorie-dense nature and the fact that we're not always aware we're consuming them. It's very rare for something to have a high protein content without you knowing about it.

Protein contains 4 calories per gram.

Now, the caveat here is that roughly a third of the calories in protein are burned in the digestion of it. So being a smartarse, you could argue that protein, in fact, only contains 2.6 calories a gram. And not only that, but it's also the most satiating, so it fills us up the most of all macronutrients, which makes it a pretty silly idea to reduce it.

We then have the requirements of protein based on our bodyweight, as mentioned earlier (see p.211). To reduce that could have a

* Metabolic syndrome: an accumulation of several disorders, which together raise the risk of an individual developing atherosclerotic cardiovascular disease, insulin resistance and diabetes mellitus.

negative impact on recovery, performance and satiety, and then put us into something called a 'negative protein balance' – this is like the calorie deficit of the protein world. If we spend too much time in a negative balance through excessive breakdown of tissues (too much training) or a lack of consumption of protein, we can then experience the opposite of MPS (muscle protein synthesis – the building process), which is muscle protein breakdown (MPB).

According to research: 'MPB is a critical aspect of the response of muscle metabolism to an exercise bout, as well as adaptations to training. Changes in the amount of any particular protein ultimately result from the balance between the rate of synthesis and breakdown of that protein over any given time.' (See References, p.288.)

So what this means is we're either technically in a building phase or a breakdown phase. The two essential players in maintaining muscle are maintaining a positive amount of protein in the diet and ensuring we're getting the right stimulus from our training.

The main reason I have explained so much about protein and dietary fats here is so that the next part makes sense.

The benefit of reducing protein to create a calorie deficit? None. It's a silly idea, which jeapordizes satiety and potentially negatively impacts on muscle mass and recovery through reducing what is, to me, the most important macronutrient. And a fun fact here: protein is derived from the Greek word *proteios*, meaning 'primary' or of most importance.

Now, the benefit of reducing fats to create a calorie deficit? Easy swaps from butters to oils, seasoning on salads or smarter food choices can mean substantial changes to the number of calories in a meal. With sensible choices, such as moving from red meat to lean meat, you may experience similar satiety, but with a reduction in calories. The main caveat is that you don't want fats to go too low, as mentioned earlier. Dietary fats are essential for not only the production of hormones, but also when consuming fat-soluble vitamins (A, D, E and K).

And the benefit of reducing carbohydrates to create a calorie deficit? An Introduction to the 'Insulin Hypothesis'.* This is where the rabbit hole begins. I feel like Morpheus in *The Matrix*, where I offer you the Red Pill or the Blue Pill. You can take the Blue Pill and we don't have to enter this chapter; you can just go on in life without having to know. But if you take the Red Pill, we're going to uncover a big subject that will liberate you with knowledge when it comes to fat loss. (See References, p.288.)

Carbohydrates (sugars and starches) are broken down into glucose, which is the body's principal and preferred energy source. It can be used immediately by the body or it can be sent to the muscles (or liver in small amounts to be stored as glycogen).

Imagine a muscle as being a bit like a battery; it has about two hours' worth of battery life (glycogen) to fuel it at any point. It's estimated that we store about this much energy (in calories) in various places:

---

* The 'insulin hypothesis' is simply where insulin is blamed for fat gain, weight gain and other detriments to our health. Low-carb zealots will proclaim you don't need to worry about calories as long as you manage your insulin. This is not factual, and when looking at a multitude of studies comparing diets with equal calories and protein we see no advantage to lower-carb conditions for fat loss.

- Muscle glycogen – 1,500kcals
- Liver glycogen – 400kcals
- Blood glucose – 80kcals
- Body fat – 80,000kcals

The body prefers to break down carbohydrates as less oxygen is required to do so compared to dietary fats or proteins. This is why in high-intensity exercise the body breaks down more carbohydrate, while we tend to use more fat as a fuel source at lower intensities. I often compare carbs/fats to an electric/petrol motor on a hybrid car. The electric (fats) are more likely to be used when manoeuvring in the big city, and then when you put your foot down on the open road, you'd switch to the petrol engine (carbohydrates). Carbohydrates are also great because they preserve muscle tissue, which is known as protein sparing.

Now, here's the bit that has turned the world on its head:

Carbohydrates, while preferred, are not essential to the human body, although protein and dietary fats are. But let's be clear that just because something is not essential it's not a reason not to include it in your life, a bit like exercise, holidays, alcohol or having a dog.

So what happens if we don't eat carbohydrates? Introducing the ketogenic diet, aka going KETO.

Does putting the majority of the population on a low-carb diet elicit fat loss through creating a deficit? YES.

Do a large number of people who do keto (which can create a calorie deficit) lose fat? YES.

Are there times and places for the strategy of the ketogenic diet to be effective for some populations? YES.

Will I ever recommend the keto diet? Fuck NO!

What is ketosis?

So when we consume food, the reason we divide it into macronutrients isn't so we become robots and see food as numbers or a colour in the pie chart on MyFitnessPal. It's so that we can understand what those foods are doing to us.

When we eat food, a small amount of breakdown can occur in the mouth. We chew and break up food for the stomach. The stomach is actually more of a preparation organ than a digestion organ, in my opinion, and it will break down foods further to pass into the small intestine, then the large intestine and then into the toilet.

Food molecules pass through the small intestine and are absorbed into the bloodstream.

Now, imagine our circulatory system as a train track: places to get on and places to get off. The lungs, for instance, are where oxygen gets on and carbon dioxide gets off. The intestines are where the nutrients get on.

Protein is broken down into amino acids in the blood – remember, these are not just required for muscle but other tissues too.

Dietary fats are broken down into fatty acids (and glycerol for you geeks reading).

Carbohydrates are broken down into glucose in the bloodstream. Pretty much sugar in the blood, circulating to be used for energy by muscles, but let's not forget the brain too. I'm sure you can remember the last time you dialled back your carbohydrates and felt a bit lethargic and like your brain was foggy.

So we have glucose circulating for when it's needed. If the amount of glucose in the blood is too high, insulin plays its part by decreasing the amount in the blood by storing it in cells. The opposing hormone is glucagon (not to be confused with glycogen), whose role it is to bring the glucose levels up when blood sugar is too low. Usually this occurs in a fasted state or prolonged period without food. (Type I diabetics – to oversimplify – do not have these mechanisms in place, so they have to manually check their blood sugar and eat carbohydrates as needed to bring their blood sugar up, or inject insulin to bring their blood sugar down.)

So, a state of ketosis is where glucose availability in the blood becomes so low that the body has to switch over to another metabolic pathway. In doing so, the body now converts fatty acids into ketones, which act in a very similar way to glucose.*

NOTE

We can enter a state of ketosis through going very low calorie, but **we can also enter a state of ketosis keeping our calories exactly the same as they are now.**

Here are two scenarios I could use to get into a state of ketosis:

Scenario 1: Keep calories the same as they are now and dial back my carbohydrates to very low amounts and my protein to moderate/low amounts.

Scenario 2: Dial back food to very low amounts, prolonged duration fasts and/or starvation.†

So why do people who try keto lose weight? These are the mechanisms:

---

* Many people who proclaim they are keto are actually not in the technical state of ketosis, they're just on a low-carb diet.

† It's possible for me to gain fat in a state of ketosis should I consume more calories than my body needs.

► They eliminate a huge number of foods from their diets – cereal, bread, pasta, sweets, fizzy drinks, biscuits, alcohol, ice cream – therefore creating a calorie deficit.

► Every 1g of carbohydrate that enters a cell requires 3g of water. Because of a drastic reduction in carbohydrates the amount of water someone holds drops too, therefore causing drastic weight reductions.

► With such a strong belief in a system and method, they adhere to the dietary guidelines better than other less restrictive diets.

► Some people anecdotally report low appetite in ketosis or low carb.

There are some people who report feeling less hungry on the ketogenic diet, but this is anecdotal and is often used as propaganda for the diet. Some people require a certain degree of 'gastric stretch' in their stomach to feel properly full, others do not. Everyone is hugely individualized when it comes to dieting, so we can't just accept 'you won't feel hungry ever' when trying to sell keto.

On the whole I find the ketogenic diet very extreme. I fully back the notion that reducing carbohydrates intermittently is a great protocol for creating a deficit. **However, to eliminate them altogether is not a good idea. Especially for those who want to perform their best.**

I've spent years teaching my clients how to diet and how to lose fat, but ideally, I want to shift them to a healthier composition where they can strive for performance goals. I think it becomes a much healthier journey and pursuit for someone when they look to increase their performance rather than their composition.

In time, I want every client to be chasing a 500m row time, a ten-rep squat max or even a complex lift. I want that to be what they think about at every meal and when they go to bed on time. We may not all be Olympic athletes in our lifetimes, but **the mindset of an aspiring athlete is much healthier than that of an aspiring dieter**. When you have lost the large majority of the fat you want to lose, I want you to become hungry for those small margins in the gym and the small margins outside of them with your work and life.

To do this, you need to consume carbohydrates, feel energized and perform your best. I didn't see any athletes make the CrossFit Games on a low-carb diet this year.

What does the science say?

I found a study in which participants were given different macronutrient splits, but the same amount of calories and protein.

'We conducted a systematic review and meta-analysis of the effects on daily energy expenditure and body fat of isocaloric diets differing in their fraction of carbohydrate to fat but with equal protein. (…) We found 32 studies representing 563 subjects matching our inclusion criteria with dietary carbohydrate ranging from 1–83 per cent and dietary fat ranging from 4–84 per cent of total calories (…) [results showed] the daily energy expenditure differences between isocaloric diets with equal protein but differing in the ratio of carbohydrate to fat. The pooled weighted mean difference in energy expenditure was 26 kcal/d greater with lower fat diets.

'**These results are in the opposite direction to the predictions of the carbohydrate-insulin model**, but the effect sizes are so small as to be physiologically meaningless. In other words, for all practical purposes "a calorie is a calorie" when it comes to body fat and energy expenditure differences between controlled isocaloric diets varying in the ratio of carbohydrate to fat.' (See References, p.288.)

To conclude, I will never be against any protocol that works for someone, but I am against this false notion that low carb is superior to other models of caloric restriction when:

- ▶ there is not enough data to support the keto diet being superior for fat loss
- ▶ there is not enough data to support the keto diet being superior for performance
- ▶ there is not enough data to support the keto diet as a sustainable solution to obesity

Should you keep the amount of protein and calories the same, if you go low-fat, high-carb OR high-fat, low-carb, it makes no difference to fat loss. This is why, in my Academy, I get my clients to aim for their calories and a protein target. The rest of the focus is on food quality and adherence because some days you may want one thing and the next day it could be different.

I believe that many consumers attribute trust to the low-carb and keto methods partly because of the use of complex language, which implies a solid scientific reasoning, even without fully understanding it themselves. On the surface, there are obvious selling points to fast drops in weight through water loss, but this can be achieved in a number of ways. The current popularity of keto diets, I believe, is because 'low-carb' has become a commonly used and well-known phrase within the diet industry. For example, although not many people in my family know what a macronutrient is, they do understand what foods 'contain carbs'.

However, your friend or family member who lost tremendous weight or fat with a low-carb diet didn't lose it because of the lower carbs; ultimately, however you spin the situation, it would have been the fact that they consumed fewer calories. The mechanisms behind low-carbohydrate or ketogenic diets remain because of the underlying principle of the calorie (fucking) deficit.

Breakfast

You're not a moped – you don't need a kickstart!

Breakfast remains a subject of confusion: people wonder, should they have it, should they not? 'James, is breakfast good?' or, 'Is it bad?' Almost like two opposing political parties you have on one side the 'Team No Breakfast' intermittent-fasting (IF) crew and on the other 'Team Breakfast'.

Team No Breakfast don't want to mess up their autophagy,* and some IF extremists will even try to insinuate that eating breakfast could be directly linked to developing cancer. Don't get me started.

The few remaining hardened soldiers of Team Breakfast will point out that it's a healthy habit and that in observational studies, people who eat breakfast are healthier. However, at this point, we should remember what was said before about those who are health seeking and who have health-seeking behaviours – that they may be more inclined to have breakfast rather than someone potentially waking up late, sleep-deprived and rushing to work.

Where do I sit?

Well, to me, a catastrophically huge question has been left out:

'What is your goal or desired outcome?'

The harsh truth is that if you're looking to lose fat, although skipping breakfast itself is not a prerequisite, it is a very handy strategy for reducing daily calories in. When we wake up a large majority of us are not

---

* Autophagy is the body's way of cleaning out dead cells. It's become a buzz word for anyone who talks about fasting. Autophagy occurs in a calorie deficit too (some will argue it only occurs fasting because of the deficit), but to be honest, it's not something you need to worry about. No one is tracking their autophagy rate on their iPhone and I guarantee an hour's extra sleep each night would give you a better return on investment.

hungry. And here are some other reasons why it's the easiest time of the day not to eat:

- Stimulating myself with coffee is a method I use to curb hunger whenever I need to, usually between the hours of 7 a.m.–2 p.m.
- Being busy or preoccupied with tasks; personally I like to get as much work done as possible first thing in the morning and food comes as an afterthought.
- It's one of the least social meals of the day, especially during the week.
- As mentioned earlier in the book, the cyclical bout of ghrelin (the hunger hormone) will soon adjust, just like it did on your last holiday, when you experienced jetlag. In time, this feeding window's requirement for food will dissipate, making it easier to skip.

NOTE

Bolstered with the knowledge from the book so far, you should understand many of the pros and cons and realize that although skipping breakfast is a good idea for fat loss, you don't need to do it every day.

The reality if you're looking to maintain or build your existing muscle mass is that it'd make sense to have breakfast. It's an opportunity to consume protein, especially if you struggle to hit your total target. It's also a feeding bout which is important for muscle building (muscle protein synthesis). So if you're someone looking to become bigger, rather than smaller, it's a good idea to see breakfast as an opportunity, rather than a prerequisite.

Why do people believe breakfast has such importance, then?

There is some interesting research into breakfast's effect on mood, behaviour and even psychology.* There are many studies into breakfast eaters having a better nutrient intake, but a fundamental caveat here is the quality of that breakfast and what they eat as opposed to just eating anything.

Some breakfast fallacies:
'Breakfast speeds up your metabolism'

This is, in fact, true, yes. However, of course your metabolism (chemical processes) is going to increase: from your mouth salivating to your throat having to push food down into your stomach and creating certain acids to break it down. Yes, there will be a significant increase in metabolism when fed vs unfed. But the real question to ask here is: 'Does that upregulation play a role in fat loss?'

And the answer to that is no. A small upregulation in metabolism does not justify a meal of several-hundred calories. It'd be the same as taking thirty steps backwards to take one forward step.

'If you skip breakfast, you'll eat more at lunch'

In a study that looked at the effects of skipping breakfast, two groups were monitored to see how not eating breakfast would affect how much food they ate at lunch. To summarise: overall, yes, skipping

---

* I prefer to leave the data alone that tries to determine breakfast's impact on mental health and mood because the impact of individual family situations and home lives are too complex to fully understand and are quite simply outside my remit as a personal trainer.

breakfast meant eating more calories at lunch. However, the net calories throughout the day as a result were still lower in the 'non-breakfast' group.

'What does the science say in combined studies?'

'The Meta-analysis of the results found a small difference in weight favouring participants who skipped breakfast. This study suggests that the addition of breakfast might not be a good strategy for weight loss, regardless of established breakfast habit. Caution is needed when recommending breakfast for weight loss in adults, as it could have the opposite effect.' (See References, p.288.)

To conclude, if you're looking to lose body fat, not eating breakfast is a good plan – not essential, but on the whole, a good, proven strategy to help you reduce calorie intake.

To flip that, if you're looking to gain weight, it'd be a good approach to eat it.

Clean eating

The clean-eating movement isn't as bad as many of the others that have passed through over time. It's just a bit daft, but it still requires a discussion. After reading this, you'll be in a position to shut down any argument about this with good, solid advice, rather than them expecting to just 'eat clean'.

So what is 'clean eating'?

Clean eating is a blanket term that often refers to wholefood eating – essentially, where you eliminate all processed foods and only eat what are considered 'single-ingredient' foods. This usually means packaged foods are forbidden, as is anything processed, such as mince, pasta and breads, and foods that have added sugar, salt or fat are dialled back too. Clean eating also promotes cooking more at home. This all sounds great and you might be wondering why there isn't a whole chapter on it in this book. You're probably thinking, James, what is your beef with clean eating?

It's all subjective, that's what my beef is!

Subjective: adjective – based on or influenced by personal feelings, tastes or opinions.

Ask ten people what clean eating is and you could have ten different responses, and they could all be correct. Clean eating is what it is to them – it doesn't have a clearly defined set of rules or structure.

You are very unlikely to visit your GP to ask for diet advice and be given a pamphlet about clean eating. And if you were, I'd be pretty pissed off.

Although I strongly agree with some of the outcomes of clean eating, it's an unhelpful way to dress up a nutritional scheme or strategy. You could easily decide to eat a grapefruit for breakfast, a bowl of organic rice for lunch and then an apple, a vegetable soup for dinner. That'd be such a clean day of eating! No processed foods, no packaged foods and you could prepare it all at home.

However, if you were to continue with that diet, you'd face all sorts of deficiencies, and if your goal was fat loss, muscle growth or recomposition, there's no dietary structure in place to suit those goals. You can eat clean with no guarantee of a deficit, a surplus or adequate protein, which is essential for a myriad reasons for performance, health and composition.

Could we do with more fruits and vegetables, to cook more and reduce the amount of processed foods? Yes. Is this the right strategy? No. And here's why.

▶ It's an extremist approach to improving the quality of the diet. Although I'm sure that it's going to be a lot more difficult to consume a hypercaloric diet when striving to 'eat clean', and it should improve the chances of someone transitioning to a hypocaloric diet (a calorie deficit), I still feel that one huge factor is left out – and that is adherence and sustainability.

I've worked with CEOs, corporate warriors, stay-at-home parents and students who were all kinds of different people, and I've never given the advice of 'just eat cleaner'. I'd classify that in the same way as advising 'eat less, move more' to the struggling dieter – it doesn't do enough for them.

▶ What if my client has had a sandwich every day for their lunch for fifteen years?
▶ What if my client wants to eat with their spouse each night for dinner?
▶ What if my client can't cook?

Whether the goal is to lose fat or build muscle – or both – flipping someone's diet on its head to become 'cleaner' isn't a good move. Although it may come with a plethora of benefits, such as improved nutrient intake, better digestion and a spontaneous reduction in calories, for most of the readers of this book it's an unsustainable shift from where they are at. I've said it many a time before on social media: 'A strength athlete has a goal in mind, but they are only ever looking to add 0.5kg* to the bar and they'll be happy with that increase today.'

- ► When you fuck up, which you will (because you're human), what tools are you left with? To eat cleaner? To eat super-clean?
- ► When you want to drink alcohol – how do you make room for that? How do you prepare for it or work it off?
- ► How do you quantify your success in your clean eating? A tick box at the end of the day? 'Did you eat clean today?' That'd be like running a team in a corporate office and getting them to answer the question: 'Did you work hard today?'

Although there are many benefits to take away from eating more 'clean', I can't get behind it as a strategy in itself. I think it goes without saying that we should be striving for more good-quality unprocessed foods, but we shouldn't demonize foods of convenience because they may be the underpinning factors right now in someone's diet.

Unfortunately (in my opinion), obesity is killing more people than processed or packaged foods are when managed with calorie control in mind. That's not to say they're a not huge contributor to chronic hypercaloric eating, but we must take a step back and look at a person's desired goals, outcomes, lifestyle and financial situation before attempting to clean up their diet.

What does the science say?

'While clean-eating sites continue to be a popular medium for women as they increasingly turn to non-traditional media outlets for information, dietitians and health professionals need to demonstrate leadership in correcting potential misinformation, reducing the risk of

---

* 0.5kg is the smallest disc I believe that you can get in Olympic lifting.

problematic eating and upholding evidence-based and balanced eating habits in the online space to protect the public.' (See References, p.288.)

To conclude, my message is not to tell you to eat 'dirty' as opposed to eating 'clean'. I just want to point out that this is a nuanced subject that is largely subjective to the person who implements it, and **a person could benefit much more if they understood components of their diet beyond simply labelling foods as clean vs dirty or good vs bad**.

To me there is no such thing as a bad food, just a bad diet.

Rather than categorizing things as good or bad, a better strategy would be to look for balance instead of placing blame on specific food types. And that's without getting into the implications it could have for developing orthorexia.*

So although it's crucial to eat better quality, less-processed foods and strive for more 'single ingredient' foods to fill our long-term sustainable diet to optimise our health, performance and wellbeing, I just don't feel 'clean eating' is advice that is quite good enough.

In a professional work place you're set key performance indicators and a salary, and we're given things to work towards on a daily, weekly, quarterly and yearly basis. I think we need to ensure that we do the same with our diet, and to just 'eat clean' isn't the answer.

---

* Orthorexia – an obsession with eating foods that one considers healthy.

Intermittent fasting

Intermittent fasting (IF) is the protocol of reducing your feeding window – the hours in which you eat. The main objective from this practice is to decrease the number of calories and food you consume in a given day.

Does it work? I reckon so, yeah. For the majority of people who go with the most common feeding windows of 1 to 9 p.m. there will be a reduction in the amount of food consumed each day. If you think about it in a very basic way, if someone who usually consumes three meals a day follows an intermittent fasting approach, they could reduce the number of meals they eat by a third, and therefore enjoy close to the same reduction in calories too. This could easily take a large proportion of the population from a hypercaloric (too many calories) to a hypocaloric day (not enough) – aka the calorie fucking deficit.

People think I hate intermittent fasting. I don't. And I'll even put my IF hat on and praise it, as follows.

The intermittent-fasting belief system

When someone is told, 'If you eat in this window, you'll lose fat,' they will believe it. Especially if it's sold well. Now, if that belief stops someone eating in the first half of their day to create a much-needed deficit, that's great! Not only that, but I feel a lot of people deal with hunger better with this belief. It's 10 a.m. and they're bloody starving, but instead of looking around their desk or in the fridge for something to eat, they look at their watch and say to themselves, 'Just three more hours' – and, before they know it, their hunger has dissipated.

I spoke earlier on in the book about how hunger management becomes habitualized, not only psychologically, but physiologically too. Looking at the habit cycle we could see this change:

I feel hungry –> I look in the fridge –> I eat food
Then, after implementing the IF approach:
I feel hungry –> I look at my watch –> I wait three hours

This should again reinforce the idea of the power of habits and beliefs in dieting. Just remember, you can make humans go to war for a country that doesn't physically exist, so getting them to hold off food until 1 p.m. should be a doddle in comparison.

I used to believe strongly in IF, and I even had my own theory as to why it was superior to a traditional calorie-restricted diet. I always thought of the human body as being fed or unfed. When fed, the body would use food in the digestive tract for fuel and not body fat. Fasted (or unfed), the body would turn to its substrates.

Substrates sounds complex, but imagine if you will the human body as a skeleton. Organs inside it doing all their functions. Pumping blood, breathing oxygen, creating and managing blood sugar and hormone production to make everything happy and keep it in what's known as homeostasis (a stable equilibrium).

Now, on that skeleton are fat and muscles that live on the bone and beneath the skin. Both of these CAN fuel the body should they be required to. It's hypothesized that fat contains around 3,500kcals a pound and muscle about 1,200kcals. Muscle is a much less efficient fuel source than fat because storing energy is not its job; its job is to create locomotion through shortening under contraction. Although you may not like the fact that we can lose muscle and not just fat in a deficit, it is actually pretty cool that this occurs from an evolutionary perspective, as early humans spent 99.9 per cent of their existence trying not to die from famine.

However, if you'd prefer not to lose your muscle in periods of caloric restriction, you can do two things:

▶ Consume adequate protein – stay in a positive protein balance and do not leave your body in a position where it needs to break down existing tissues for its amino-acid requirements.

▶ Train the damn things – use it or lose it, mate. Should there be no requirement for muscle or inadequate stimuli, the body will not require excess weight. It's a bit like closing the rear passenger window on a car when your mate gets out – there's no need for it to be open and, although a negligible effect, you can reduce the car's drag by winding it up closed.

So surely being in a fasted state would lead to more fat loss?

I thought so too. But no, it doesn't. It boils down to energy in vs out, I'm afraid, and IF doesn't have any tangible benefits over regular calorie restriction.

So what I'm saying is, there is no difference between consuming 2,000 calories, of which 200g are protein, between 1 and 9 p.m. or between 8 a.m. and 10 p.m.

Now, is that a reason not to do IF? No, it still works for a lot of people, and I'm not discouraging the practice. I'm just trying to educate you. But why? Because breakfast.

It's my favourite meal. I love nothing more than overpriced poached eggs on avocado and sourdough in a pretentious café in Bondi, Sydney. Although I am well aware I am more likely to sustain and adhere to a deficit in a shortened feeding window, it's sometimes better to just eat breakfast. Let's look at the repercussions too! I'm not going to visit said pretentious overpriced café and drink a black coffee only to then watch my friend eat my favourite breakfast in front of me. Why not? Because then it'd feel a lot like I am on a diet and that's not a headspace I want to be in.

I want a future where IF is a tool, not a belief. I want the flow of misinformation to stop and for people to stand on their scales, look in the mirror or even measure their waist circumferences and realize the world is not over – they have many tools as their disposal and intermittent intermittent fasting is a good idea for them to create a deficit and drop any unwanted body fat.

Yeah, I just made that up – the James Smith way, of course.

Intermittent intermittent fasting = occasionally skipping fucking breakfast for fat loss, mate

So what misinformation is out there with regard to intermittent fasting?

Don't you burn more fat when you fast for a longer period?

We saw this previously with fasted cardio – keep in mind too that EAT (the exercise component of daily expenditure – see p.61) is merely 10 per cent in most people, so looking at our daily lives, fasted vs fed is very similar to looking at fat loss during exercise fasted vs fed.

Fat loss is not greater among those who practise IF vs non-time-restricted feeding windows. I'd advise that personal preference should always be the winner when deciding what to eat. Intermittent fasting does not benefit fat loss, but it doesn't hurt it either.

Aren't you much more alert in a fasted state?

Okay, this one I shall concede on a bit. Don't think of fasting as having clarity, but rather as feeding bringing about a post-prandial lull. It's very normal for us to feel a bit lethargic after eating and this can affect our alertness, but then often I would rather eat breakfast and have a few too many coffees than be hungry and alert.

Some theorize that the alertness comes from the body's evolutionary response to seek food. This is why I've heard reports of poor sleep from clients who go to bed hungry or are low-carb (and I know from personal experience too). This could be another benefit of IF, on reflection – that people typically are 'allowed' to have larger feedings before they go to sleep at night, so not only are they feeling more alert during the day, they may feel more tired at night, which then leads to an earlier bed time, better-quality sleep, etc.

I used to nap around lunchtime or early afternoon when I was doing one-to-one PT, so I'd have a meal beforehand to help me sleep. There is no wrong or right here, and some people who work in an office may only be permitted to eat lunch at a specified time. It wouldn't be feasible for them to say, 'Oh, I have to wait until 1 p.m.'

You could eat 12–8 p.m., 11 a.m.–7 p.m. or any time of the day, as long as you hit the same number of calories.

Autophagy

Most of the debate with regard to this subject surrounds the pronunciation of the bloody word. I say *autof-agey*; some others say *auto-fay-gee*. Who is right? No one seems to know. It's like the wonderful town of Cairns in Australia. Some call it *canz*, others pronounce it *care-nz*.

But more importantly – what is it? Autophagy, which we touched on earlier in the breakfast section of the book, is an evolutionary breaking-down process by which cells degrade and recycle on an intracellular level.

A bloke named Yoshinori won a Nobel Prize in 2016 for making clear the role of autophagy in the human body. (It's actually crazy that some people use this as an argument in their debate for fasting: 'Well, James, if it's not that significant, why did someone get a Nobel Prize for discovering and clarifying the mechanism?'

It's theorized that dysfunctional autophagy can contribute to a lot of diseases, including cancer. It's also theorized that autophagy can play a role in preventing cancer, but there just isn't enough strong evidence, I feel, to say that for sure. However, in the last few years autophagy has become a trigger word, and some zealots now proclaim fasting is a cure for cancer and can help you live longer. I think we should all look beyond our feeding windows when examining factors that influence life expectancy – to things like sleep, sunlight, nutrition, socioeconomic status, training, etc. – not the fact that Bill lived to 121 years old because he fucking skipped breakfast.

According to research, '… both fasting and calorie restriction have a role in the upregulation of autophagy, the evidence overwhelmingly suggesting that autophagy is induced in a wide variety of tissues and organs in response to food deprivation.' (See References, p.288.)

I wasn't even going to talk about autophagy in this book, and I've never had a client who moved their feeding windows or decreased calories and came in with a spring in their step because of autophagy, nor have any of my clients ever reported noticing more cell recycling occurring. Our focus needs to be on our efforts and practices on a daily basis, and if that means increases in autophagy happen off the back of it, so be it. However, we should not be getting too caught up on our feeding windows, but should instead focus on the most sustainable way to create a deficit for fat loss. Seeing as both caloric restriction AND fasting periods can have a role in upregulation of autophagy, we can therefore pick which one favours our lifestyle best.

To conclude, until we have an app on the iPhone that notes our levels of autophagy (however it's bloody pronounced), I think we have more important things to be concerned with at this moment in time, don't you?

Training vs exercising

What I want to clarify in this section of the book are what I deem to be the differences between training and exercising. These are my own personal opinions, so don't expect a study to back my ramblings.

Exercising

This is any training that sits within the EAT category. Should you stand on the Tube or take the stairs, let's not get it twisted – that's NEAT not EAT (see p.61 for more on these).

Walking or plodding on a treadmill or cross-trainer I consider exercise – it's a means of increasing the amount of calories burned in a day within a set time frame, but there's not often a 'plan' in place to achieve a certain result or train a certain muscle.

Exercise is often ad hoc and done in varying amounts with little consistency, and usually upregulated in periods of over-indulgence.

We are a walking, talking, breathing encapsulation of our daily eating, drinking and exercise habits.

Training

Training, to me, is having a goal and making our way towards it with a plan of action and steps in place to progress. Remember that people often have similar goals – just not everyone follows a plan or process to get to them. That's what distinguishes people who accomplish their goals from those who don't.

Training requires and demands a specific outcome from the time spent training, whether at home or at the gym.

Let's look at compositional goals:

- **To be leaner** This requires a calorie deficit over time.
- **To be more muscular** This is training with the objective of muscle growth – or hypertrophy. This requires progressive overload, which I'll talk about shortly. Also, there is a requirement for the right amount of calories and protein.
- **To be more defined** This would be a combination of both simultaneously. Muscle growth can and does occur in people who are dieting to be leaner, but dieting can hinder results. Imagine if you will, a rugby player who wants to be stronger and faster. He can't be out on the track and lifting weights in the same session. Should he want to focus on more speed he may have to swap some of his strength sessions if he's limited in how many times he can train a day.

Then we have performance goals:

- A personal best (PB) lift
- A technical movement performed well, like a snatch or muscle up
- Time over distance – for instance, a 500m row or a 5k run

Now, I will *always* opt for my clientele to aim for the latter and set a performance-based goal because I truly don't think seeking just low body-fat/composition goals are healthy for the body or the mind long-term. Wherever or whatever your fitness journey, there is someone out there who will look better, I'm sorry to say. Just as no matter how rich you are, someone out there is richer. You could buy the biggest fuck-ing yacht in the world, but I promise you one day you'll park in a harbour next to a bigger one.

If you're obese, then the initial part of your journey must be finding a sustained path to no longer being that way. For the majority of people who are obese, this doesn't even need to be in the gym. I did a TV show with a lovely lady I was partnered up with to help her lose weight over a month. I remember asking her, 'Do you like the gym?' She responded, 'I see a PT twice a week.' I assumed from how she dodged answering the actual question that perhaps the gym wasn't a place she wanted to spend a lot of time in, so I gave her 10,000 steps a day and 1,600 calories. She dropped 7.5kg in just over three weeks without having to go to the gym. In time she will be ready to set her first performance goal and, from there, the physique that comes with it will be more of a by-product of striving for that goal, rather than a goal in itself.

With social media we are exposed to an array of physiques like never before. When we look at the compositional goals, they are very one-dimensional: eat less and move weights through the same plane of motion and repeat and repeat until you're happy with how you look. *Spoiler alert:* which is usually never.

What if I said to you that 0.00001 per cent of the world has perfect genetics. Perfect, out-of-this-world genetics. Of course, I am making this up to prove a point, but just imagine that for a second. Now, what are the chances of you bumping into that person at Westfield shopping centre? What are the chances of you knowing them? However, with modern-day social media, you'd have over 775 people to choose from to follow on Instagram today with that percentile of the world's entire population.

Performance goals are where it is at! Not just for your gym training, but your peace of mind. This is one of the reasons CrossFit has done so well over the years, putting the community aspect aside. Trisha from Northampton is working towards her first set of five unassisted chin ups rather than comparing her stomach to someone of her age on the front cover of *Women's Health* mag.

I find it healthy for both genders in different ways, as opposed to the majority of men who try to go down a bodybuilder 'bro' route where bigger is better. I have been there myself – and it's usually whoever is willing to do the most anabolic steroids who comes out on top: big arms, big chest, massive shoulders. Not only is it unobtainable for a lot of people, but you have corporate blokes who have an hour a day to train comparing themselves to a lad ten years younger who trains full time and has all of his meals sent to him.

I take so much pleasure in knowing that someone out there, let's call him Steve, has just got his first muscle up, his hands are sore and he has chalk all over him. He's been turning up day in, day out trying to master the technical feat of his first muscle up. He will go home, his wife will be so happy he has done so well and they can both rejoice in his progression without him having to take his top off and find immaculate lighting.

I speak from experience of being someone who strived for the bodybuilder physique. I succumbed to anabolic steroids – and for what? Trying to fit in or keep up with the other men I saw on social media: totally not worth it. I was much happier with my own first muscle up than I was at the end of twelve-week cycle of anabolics.

Now, in recent years we have seen a huge transformation in female physique training, and I must credit one of my most influential mentors here, Bret Contreras. Bret invented the barbell hip thrust, which is a movement primarily recruiting the hip joint and driven by the glutes (which means bum muscles). Until recently, female physiques have not had much of a direction to go in, with the thinking being that a good set of shoulders is 'bulky' or muscular thighs or arms being 'masculine'. In recent years, we have seen a growing movement of women training and focusing on hypertrophy, primarily for their bum and hamstrings. And I'm not even speculating – I'm telling you for a fact that this movement has liberated hundreds of thousands of women with a training direction that they actually want and can sustain.

Over the last few years, it's been great to see women coming into gyms and setting up their barbell hip thrusts, as men look over wondering how on earth they're lifting so much. They've been at it a while, they have a goal and they're coming in each day to accomplish it. Humans need a sense of purpose – it's why religions and other beliefs are so popular. But I feel we especially need it when it comes to training. We're often not motivated by the health benefits associated with training, and a lot of the time we need to be inching towards a goal or some form of progress. Those who are training (as opposed to those who are exercising) are striving for what is known as 'progressive overload'.

What is 'progressive overload'?

Progressive overload is quite simply about doing more, but in a more objective than subjective manner. It's hard to say, 'Oh, you need to be increasing your squat by 1kg every seven days', because there are so many factors at play in every scenario.

So first of all you need a starting point, which depends on who walks through the door when I am personal training. If my mum came in, I'd probably get her to sit on a bench or box similar to what she's familiar with to find a comfortable starting point to progress from, perhaps the sofa. (She'd note it's a bit easier than usual because she'd be doing it without the glass of wine!) I could get her to sit down and stand back up ten times.

I'd then ask her how hard she found it out of ten. This is known as rate of perceived exhaustion (RPE), and it's what I use with all my James Smith Academy members to keep them on top of their progressive-overload needs. She'd sit down and stand back up, then say to me that it 'feels like an eight or nine out of ten difficulty'.

Progressive overload for my mum could be to increase her reps. If, in a few weeks' time, she can do eighteen reps before it's perceived as an eight or nine out of ten, she has accomplished progressive overload. From here, there are many ways for me to adapt her training. I could:

- ► give her a weight to hold
- ► slow down her lowering sit
- ► lower the box height
- ► bring in a pause or a quarter rep.

As you can see there are plenty of ways to skin a cat – that was me just naming a few from the off. If you left me to train my mum for several weeks, when you came back she might have progressed to a barbell for ten reps without the requirement for a box. That's not exercising; that's training – and without chasing anything unobtainable, only to progressively overload the exercise she was already doing. See someone in the gym with a big lift? Guess what – they progressively overloaded their way there, whether they know it or not.

The experience of the person lifting will determine which methods are used to increase progressive overload. For instance, a more experienced lifter may even say they're trying to break a plateau while attempting progressive overload.

This is what Bret says:

After proper form and full range of motion are established and ingrained, now it's time to worry about progressing in repetitions and load. But these aren't the only ways to progress. Here are all the practical ways I can think of:

- Lifting the same load for increased distance (range of motion)
- Lifting the same load and volume with better form, more control and less effort (efficiency)/Lifting the same load for more reps (volume)
- Lifting heavier loads (intensity of load)
- Lifting the same load and volume with less rest time in between sets (density)
- Lifting a load with more speed and acceleration (intensity of effort)
- Doing more work in the same amount of time (density)
- Doing the same work in less amount of time (density)
- Doing more sets with the same load and reps (volume)
- Lifting the same load and volume more often throughout the week (frequency)
- Doing the same work while losing body mass (increased relative volume)
- Lifting the same load and volume and then extending the set past technical failure with forced reps, negatives, drop sets, static holds, rest pause, partial reps or post-exhaustion (intensity of effort)

Just remember, improvements in form and range of movement come first, and increases in reps and load come second.*

I personally feel that this growing movement of aspiring to have well-developed legs is fantastic because so many of my clients and other people's clients are working towards progressing their big

* Bret Contreras @bretcontreras1

compound lifts, and hip thrusts have become the nucleus of their regime. This is a positive movement because this isn't just for appearance; it's for performance, strength increases, and going to the gym with a goal that goes beyond just wanting to look better.

To conclude, having sights set on progression and progressive overload should be the key focal point for someone who is either new to training or has lost the amount of fat they want to lose. Transitioning from obese should not be directed towards very defined abs and a six-pack; it should be about getting in shape, so that you can start working your arse off towards a performance-based goal that you will, in time, accomplish, and then setting the bar slightly higher.

That concludes the difference between training and exercising. Big credit to Bret Contreras for all he has done for the world of lifters, especially for those who are female and now find themselves with a strong direction that doesn't involve starving themselves to fit in. Progressive overload is a goal that is never fully met, and that's what makes it a great focus for those who are training with intent. That is why you can't just exercise and expect a training response.

Female Fat Loss

Rewind a couple of years and I was waking up at 4.45 a.m. to get from Bondi, Sydney, to the Central Business District, where I worked in a Fitness First. My first client would be at 6 a.m., so I needed to wake up, hop on the train and do my 'LIVE' video on Facebook. For a long time, I couldn't really afford a fancy camera or a new laptop; and I didn't know how to edit, so I just pressed 'go live' and I'd answer people's questions as they came in. It became a ritual, and each day I'd go live without fail. When the Australia daylight savings kicked in, a 5.30 live was 8.30 p.m. in the UK.

I'd set up in a food court called 'Australia Square', and we'd joke about how the floor cleaners would always turn their machines on as soon as I started answering questions. Most questions I answer are the same every single day. People often ask if I get fed up of being asked the same questions day in and day out, and the answer is of course not. I don't think anyone out there is asking for the sake of it; they're not getting a kick out of me repeating myself. It's hundreds of individuals, even thousands, who ask, then go away with more knowledge than they had before. We all repeat ourselves in our different lines of work; no one truly has something different every day. A barista makes the best coffee he can, but there are only so many combinations, and although people walk away happier and caffeinated, I like to think I can offer more – not just knowledge, but liberation.

So there I was, reeling off the answers to questions, then one hit me right in the face, and for the first time in weeks I had no idea how to answer it: 'James, do you know how our menstrual cycle affects our diet and our training?'

Long pause … 'No.'

I was preoccupied with this question for the entire duration of my 6 a.m. client. I thought to myself, James, mate, you have pretty much only trained females for nearly three years – how do you not know this? I googled some stuff at lunch, then looked for podcasts, books, whatever I could find to upskill myself on the menstrual cycle and how it affects female physiology. The rabbit hole went deeper than a clown's pocket. It used to take me about thirty minutes to get home from the CBD after work, and I found myself taking longer and longer routes to try to learn what I could.

I came to realize that I'd uncovered a very big flaw in my own personal training. I was training women simply as smaller men. This did not stem from a consciously patriarchal or misogynistic mindset; I quite simply never knew how the variable factors around the menstrual cycle could affect a woman's diet and training.

On the floor, with my clients, I'd had many conversations I didn't expect – topics ranging from infidelity, wealth, professional life, unprofessional life and even anal sex – but never had the subject of periods really come up. If it had, I'd probably have been very confused as to why and changed the subject to 'how hard is that out of ten?' – the rate of perceived exertion saving me from having to talk about 'that time of the month'.

If I were to give an elevator pitch on female physiology now, I'd say this:

A woman's physiology is unique because it is solely responsible for the survival of the human race. Women get pregnant whereas men do not. Because of this, women must store body fat in a 'readiness' state for getting pregnant between the years of the first menstruation (adolescence) to the last (menopause). It's estimated that a woman will require 50,000 calories' worth of stores to survive the duration of pregnancy, so dieting a woman is much different to dieting a man.

Men burn calories quicker than women. If a couple go to dinner and have the same burger and chips (where calories are matched), then the next day they go to burn that number of calories 'off', they would lose the same amount of fat in theory. However, it would take the woman about a third longer to do so. This means the woman having to train for ninety minutes as opposed to the man's sixty-minute workout.

Not only this, women 'push back' a lot harder during periods of extreme food restriction from a physiological as well as a psychological perspective. That's without mentioning their menstrual cycle.

The menstrual cycle

Let's see the cycle as the length or period of time between the first menstruation (bleeding) and the next. And let's imagine this occurs on the first day of the month, to make things easier, especially for any men reading.

Let's say this cycle is twenty-eight days (usually a normal cycle is twenty-five to thirty days – anything longer could be an underlying sign of PCOS, which I'll get on to a little later).

In the middle we have ovulation – this is where the eggs are released from the ovaries, therefore making this the most fertile phase for pregnancy to occur. The period leading up to this middle point is known as the follicular phase.

It's interesting to note that during ovulation – around Day 13 or 14 of their cycle – women have their highest amount of testosterone, which

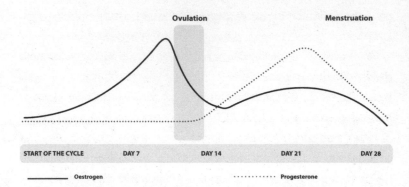

plays a large part in libido and sex drive. I've heard from my female clients over the years that they report being hornier during this period, and also manage some of their best lifts/performances. It makes complete sense from an evolutionary perspective to have a heightened sex drive at this time, so that the chances of pregnancy are increased. Men do have ten to thirty times more testosterone than women, but I've dated quite a few girls where you'd think that statistic was the other way round come the middle of their cycle.

Let's take a quick glance at the first part of the cycle, the **follicular phase, approximately** Days 1–14. Looking at the diagram, you'll notice that oestrogen is the dominant hormone on this side. (In some literature you'll see it called oestradiol.) Over the years, oestrogen has been blamed for a lot of things, and it's almost been seen as a 'bad hormone' for things like skin and water retention. But oestrogen actually has proved helpful with muscle soreness in studies, and there is now a large body of research into its impact on improving insulin sensitivity. When oestrogen drops significantly during menopause, which I'll discuss a little later, people can run into a lot of trouble trying to lose fat with lower levels of it.

I've found over the years that my clientele respond better to training, find technical lifts the easiest, and mood, morale and adherence to dietary protocols much easier before and during ovulation.

Now, without sounding pessimistic, after ovulation, things … well, they feel like they go to shit. Welcome to the **luteal phase:** the second half of the menstrual cycle. This phase is typically fourteen days long in most women.

Hunger cravings usually shoot up in this second half, and it's believed this is due to women's metabolic rate increasing their calorie needs by around 100–300kcals a day. Some women find themselves consuming about 500kcals more a day. With cravings in mind, for my James Smith Academy members I factor in some extra fruit during this part of the cycle. Easy, convenient, cheap and socially acceptable to eat on a train, Tube or even in a meeting, fruit can have a massive impact on hunger cravings, especially when you want something sweet. You could easily have three pieces of fruit a day just to match the increase in your metabolic rate.

In the luteal and progesterone-dominant part of the menstrual cycle we see a rise in insulin resistance, a decrease in performance and even a higher chance of dislocation and injury. If you're a man reading this and you have to compete in a sport on a certain date, just realize how lucky you are that you don't have to worry about where you are in your cycle. Men have pretty much the same physiology every day of the month, and the only decline that's noted is related to ageing (or lack of sleep, remember?). But some women note that their performance lifts are half what they were a week before. Following on from progressive overload, we must take into consideration how deflating this could be for someone whose plan doesn't take this into consideration, or if a trainer lacks the necessary empathy for fluctuations in performance related to the menstrual cycle.

Since learning about this and continuing to have in-depth conversations with my female clientele and members, I often get them to look at their training programmes, keeping in mind that sometimes adjustments need to be made on the exercises: a squat may become a leg press; a bent over row may become a TRX row; I'll move them on to more machines instead of free weights; and I will make sure they're fully prepared to go into the gym not expecting miracles or personal bests. They're fighting their physiology in this period and the last thing they need are high expectations on their performance when, quite simply, they're not going to get them.*

Here are some important strategies that I implement with my female clients:

- ▶ Measuring progress week on week for every cycle, rather than week to week consecutively. Week 1 vs Week 3 can be two hugely different places in the cycle, so the readings would not be accurate. Even weighing and measuring on the same day each week may not fit into the menstrual cycle's rotation. So if you take measurements, keep them as consistent as possible. By this I mean you should compare your measurements from week one of one cycle to week one of the next, and so on. Measure at menstruation, measure at ovulation, but keep it consistent.
- ▶ Starting a dieting phase. The follicular phase (the one–two weeks at the start of your cycle) is always going to be the best time to implement caloric restriction or a new training

* For detailed instruction on every gym and home-based exercise visit www.jamessmithacademy.com.

cycle. Implementing it just after ovulation could spell disaster with adherence and leave women feeling very deflated.

▶ During the period of premenstrual syndrome (PMS) symptoms (usually the one–two weeks at the end of your cycle) increase food intake slightly – three pieces of fruit or something similar. Play around with it and see what works for you.

▶ Not dieting every week. Lots of the women I train only diet for the first two weeks of their cycle. They can then sit at maintenance rather than deficit for the latter two weeks (luteal). This isn't for everyone, but aggressive dieting for two weeks of the month typically works better long-term than yo-yo silly dieting with no efficacy. So if you wish to only diet for two weeks of each month as a strategy, that is completely fine and something I urge you to try out yourself. Each woman needs to be her own scientist with all of this. There are good times to diet and also not so good times, and it is your prerogative to restrict when you can and to eat normally when you can't.

I find that the use of performance-enhancing drugs is rife in everything from the Olympics to amateur sports, not to mention the regular gym goer, and they're very popular with women too. This not only increases their performance and speeds up their recovery, but allows them to manipulate their cycle around their competing days, especially in sports like Olympic lifting, where you need to be in peak condition.

I don't condone the use of performance-enhancing drugs in sporting events like the Olympics, but I do sympathize with having to deal with managing cycles for performance.

If you think about the difference across most disciplines between fourth and first place, it can sometimes be fractions of a second. Some women report up to a 40 per cent decrease in strength during their luteal phase, and I know that intentional amenorrhoea (discontinuation of the menstrual cycle) is a tactic some women who compete use, while others prefer dieting past the point of amenorrhoea, as their cycle doesn't affect them as much.

Amenorrhoea

The absence of menstruation in a female between the reproductive ages of approximately twelve and forty-nine years old for ninety days or more is known as amenorrhoea. (Oligomenorrhoea is an infrequent or irregular cycle at intervals of greater than thirty-five days, with only four to nine periods in a year.)

This can happen for different reasons. When testing someone to determine why, you can use the following methods:

- ▶ Pregnancy test – pregnancy being the most common cause of amenorrhoea
- ▶ Testosterone and DHEAS (a male sex hormone found in men and women) to rule out hyperandrogenism*
- ▶ BMI (to look for malnutrition, anorexia nervosa and excessive strenuous exercise)

* Hyperandrogenism is a medical condition characterized by high levels of androgens (known as 'male hormones', but also present in females). Symptoms may include acne, inflamed skin, hair loss on the scalp, increased body or facial hair and infrequent or lack of menstruation. This is one of the three contributors towards a diagnosis of PCOS (see opposite page).

Most of the cases of amenorrhoea I have come across are to do with a lack of calories or excessive and strenuous exercise. I am not a doctor, nor am I qualified in this field, but I have learned a lot from my research and from talking to my many female clients about their menstrual cycles – or lack thereof.

I think it goes without saying that not having enough calories in your diet or being too lean could make someone not want to get pregnant, due to the fact that they may not be able to sustain the pregnancy. In the same way that if you're skint, you're more likely to say no to a night out with your friends, so to speak. Also, if strenuous exercise is a contributor to the excessive deficit or low body-fat percentages, then perhaps doing less exercise would be a good solution to lower the deficit or to make more calories available for functions such as the reproductive system.

Please seek medical advice if you are concerned about this condition.

PCOS

PCOS – or polycystic ovary syndrome – affects around 10 per cent of women, and is another very common reason for amenorrhoea. It is also associated with infertility. Around 20 per cent of females who struggle to get pregnant are diagnosed with PCOS.

Polycystic ovary syndrome ties in with amenorrhoea because from my own experience training women they can often come hand in hand. Those with PCOS can suffer with amenorrhea and vice versa. PCOS is correlated with weight gain, which I'll expand on, but from what I know, weight loss between someone who has PCOS and a female who doesn't can differ, should their deficit be the same.

The criteria for diagnosing PCOS are:

- ▸ Polycystic ovaries – having physical cysts on your ovaries
- ▸ Oligomenorrhoea/amenorrhoea (see p.268)
- ▸ Hyperandrogenism (see p.268)

If you have two of these, you're classified as having PCOS, so what does that mean for most?

- ▸ Increased risk of Type II diabetes
- ▸ Insulin resistance
- ▸ Increased risk of cardiovascular disease
- ▸ Infertility and pregnancy complications

PCOS is more prevalent in the overweight, and exercise and weight loss, just like with Type II diabetes, have been proven to improve it. Martin MacDonald (a mentor, peer and friend), who I learned a lot of this from, made a great point when he said that although you could argue this is outside the scope of what a PT has to deal with, where else can we direct people? See a doctor? Most people report to us that they're not happy with their doctors. Same goes for dietitians – what if their rubbish doctor refers them to a rubbish dietitian? Not only that, but often the very good dieticians and doctors are full, because they're good. It's a vicious circle. Exercise and weight loss are key factors in improving the symptoms of PCOS, and both are things that personal trainers are qualified to do, so I'll carry on.

The insulin resistance part of the problem is worth talking about because it can often be left unexplained during diagnosis of PCOS. So insulin resistance (IR) leads to increased blood glucose and/or increased blood insulin levels (hyperinsulinemia). This then worsens the androgen profile (see footnote on p.268) for women, which leads to increased levels of testosterone.

Whether it's Type II diabetes or PCOS, the objective must be about increasing insulin sensitivity – the opposite of insulin resistance. The main and best way to do this is to decrease total body fat through implementing a calorie deficit alongside training and being active. Training a muscle makes the muscle more insulin-sensitive, which is another reason I would always advise weight training for women with PCOS (or even without), not to mention combining that with all you have learned so far in this book.

Fat gain is a protective mechanism: it's there to save us not just in the future, but right now too. You can hear about diabetics losing their eyesight and damaging vessels to the point of losing limbs. Too much glucose in the blood will cause damage, so having fat cells to soak up excess 'energy' in the blood is a great mechanism to protect us. *When we become resistant to this process, however, damage begins to occur and we start to see a deterioration in our health. Too much of anything in life will start to affect our health and fat is one of those.*

Key PCOS facts

- ▶ Muscles become more insulin-sensitive after training them – another reason to resistance train.
- ▶ A lot of people hypothesize that carbs = insulin, therefore = don't have carbs. That's not the case. Maybe a slight reduction in carbs is needed to create the necessary calorie deficit, but all in all, total fat loss is the key driver, coupled with resistance training to improve overall insulin sensitivity.
- ▶ Not all people with PCOS have IR.

- Striving for a 'low-GI'* diet can help symptoms and improve quality of life.
- High protein diets recommended (2g per kg+ is my personal recommendation for satiety and other complex reasons associated with PCOS), due to their ability to also aid with weight maintenance.
- Stress management is not only important before implementing caloric restriction, but needs extra attention when going head to head with any complicated syndrome such as PCOS.
- Those with PCOS register up to a 14 per cent lower BMR (= calories burned at rest) – and a huge 40 per cent lower BMR has been reported in women with both **PCOS and insulin resistance**.

Something quite powerful here is that even if you're a male and you're still reading this far or you're a fortunate female who doesn't suffer with these issues, you're literally in a position of power to help and to educate those around you. Without sounding like I am attacking dieticians or the health system, pointing your friends to these pages could not only be a cost-effective means, but also give them the evidence-based advice that they currently don't have.

Supplementation for PCOS:

- **Vitamin D supplementation** has been shown to decrease the prevalence of Type II diabetes and increase insulin sensitivity.

* GI stands for glycaemic index, which is how fast blood glucose rises after consuming food. The GI rating is scored 1–100, which represents the rise of glucose in the blood two hours after food. Avoiding junk food, sweets, etc. can help with this.

You can get tested for Vitamin D deficiencies at GPs, but this can be expensive. If you suspect you have inadequate Vitamin D, try supplementing or aiming for more sunlight.

▸ **Inositol supplementation.** A recent meta-analysis of Inositol showed to be effective in promoting ovulation in patients with PCOS. It revealed that inositol (or myo-inositol) alone improves the metabolic profile of women with PCOS. (See References, p 288.)

People who suffer with PCOS could potentially be eating what is considered very few calories – say, 1,200 calories each day – and not be losing body fat. In these instances, you should consider trying some out-of-the-box methods, such as full-day fasts – even two-day fasts – and an adaptive 5:2 style of dieting, where you fast for two days a week. This is in order to create a substantial deficit on those days, and then eating would seem a lot more normal on the others, but overall your calories over a week would be lower.

When someone knows the regular amount of food they should eat on a 'normal day' (maintenance calories), you could implement alternate day fasts based on this amount, which may be easier to adhere to compared with eating half the 'normal' amount every day.

Please note, I wouldn't usually implement such restrictive protocols, but in some PCOS cases, especially with insulin resistance, it's essential for fat loss.*

When in doubt always speak to your doctor or medical professional.

---

* A special mention here to Martin MacDonald and his MNU for helping me fully understand the roles of insulin resistance and PCOS.

Menopause

Menopause: the period in a woman's life when menstruation ceases.

Roughly half the planet will at some point go through the menopause, so it's worth talking about.

For any parent it becomes quite obvious when your child hits puberty and they experience drastic changes in their physiology, mood, growth, etc. Parents are clued up quite well: they know their daughter will start menstruating and they know their son's balls are going to drop and their voice too. I remember when I was about ten or eleven, I got a cold, my dad told me my voice had dropped and I told him it was just the cold. Three months later, he said to me, 'Son, your voice hasn't gone back to what it was before'. Only there and then did I realize it had, in fact, dropped. Within the next year, I grew about a foot and became one of the largest guys in my school.

That's the first part of the picture as far as hormones and physiology are concerned. The latter part is not discussed, nor have any of my female clientele really ever been educated about what is going to happen to their bodies as they get older – when, effectively, their reproductive systems shut down and the associated hormones take a dive, causing a myriad of issues that just aren't spoken about enough within the fitness industry.

After I'm roughly thirty my testosterone will decline at a rate of about 1 per cent each year. I can influence this a bit with good sleep, good diet and sunlight exposure and looking after myself. (Oh, sorry – you already know this, as you've read this far in the book. I do apologize!) However, a woman's hormones will pretty much shut down as she approaches menopause.

The menopause most commonly occurs when a woman is in her fifties (the average age is fifty-one), but can happen earlier, in the forties, and I've even had clients who have gone through it in their thirties, some due to specific circumstances and others not. A hysterectomy, where the womb and sometimes other parts of the reproductive system are removed, will lead to a state very similar to the menopause. A lot of women will end up doing hormone replacement therapy (HRT) to relieve the symptoms of menopause. For more information **and to decide whether or not to consider it, you should talk to a medical professional**.

The repercussions of having your reproductive hormones discontinue are usually hot flushes, mood swings, trouble sleeping and changes in fat distribution to the midsection. You need a discontinuation of menstruating for twelve months to be in a state of menopause, and the discontinuation occurs due to a lack of production of oestrogen.

The first signs of menopause are in the phase known as **perimenopause**, or PM ('peri', meaning surrounding, close or near). Perimenopause is a transitionary state from menstruating to no longer menstruating. For some it can last years, and for others only months. The common symptoms are a decline in libido, trouble sleeping, hot flushes and moodiness. From a hormonal standpoint, this is very much like the follicular phase (first half of the menstrual cycle – see p.264), and oestrogen is dominant – it's usual for people to report PMS being less severe in this period too.

Towards the end of PM, the woman's physiology will begin to shift towards more of a progesterone-dominant profile, which is more indicative of menopause beginning. The hormonal profile here is similar to the luteal phase (second half of the menstrual cycle – see p.265). After this occurs, and when there's been no period for twelve months, the woman is now officially in menopause. There can be changes in body-fat distribution, weight gain, muscle loss and sometimes reports of becoming insulin resistant in this period.

Breastfeeding and pregnancy calories

It's very important that I put in this book how important nutrition is not only during and after pregnancy, but even before someone becomes pregnant – for the woman's health and the health of the baby. The composition of the woman during and before pregnancy can cause issues, so striving for a healthy weight before conceiving should be a priority. Training during pregnancy is a recommended practice, but ensure that especially in the second and third trimester, you are mindful of what exercises you are doing. I always advise pre- and post-natal women to seek advice from a pre-/post-natal specialist during training.

'Caloric intake should increase by approximately 300 kcal/day during pregnancy. This value is derived from an estimate of 80,000 kcal needed to support a full-term pregnancy. (…) However, energy requirements are generally the same as for non-pregnant women in the first trimester, increasing in the second trimester. Furthermore, energy requirements vary significantly, depending on a woman's age, BMI and activity level. Caloric intake should therefore be individualized based on these factors.' (See References, p.288.)

With regards to changes in calories required during pregnancy, this is a question I get asked a lot. My advice is always to seek advice from a medical professional, but these are the nutrition guidelines I've found:

'Women who breastfeed require approximately 500 additional kcal/day. (…) During pregnancy, most women store an extra 2 to 5kg (19,000 to 48,000kcal) in tissue, mainly as fat, in physiologic preparation for lactation. If women do not consume the extra calories, then body stores are used to maintain lactation. It is not unusual for lactating women to lose 0.5–1.0kg/month after the first postpartum month.' (See References, p.288.)

When it comes to supplementing during the planning and/or pregnancy phase, I'd recommend folic acid and Vitamin D, not to mention working closely alongside a doctor or specialist.

I've included this section in the book as I have witnessed how the knowledge does not just have an impact on how I am with my clients, but how my clients are with themselves. I've got the feeling that, for years, women have been frustrated, confused and unaware of the implications of their physiology on their ability to lose fat and maintain training performance. Being armed with the knowledge of knowing when it's good to diet and when it's not so good; preparing for sessions that will be suboptimal; and planning the sessions where you go for a personal best: all these things play a significant role in how women can feel about themselves and their attitudes towards their diet and training.

I wanted to put this in the book for men to read too. In comparison to women's, our physiology is only really influenced by age, and we need to not only have a basic understanding of how women's bodies differ to our own, but be able to empathize with that – especially if we are the ones implementing a training plan for them. Whether you're a personal trainer, brother, son or husband, it's important to take some of this upon yourself to realize not everyone has it as good as us!

Understanding these things will mean liberation and empowerment for every reader. I want every woman to walk away and be their very own scientist moving forward, armed with the confidence to query the next diet or training advice they see, and empowered to continue educating themselves with the foundations I have set, trialling what works for them and discovering ultimately what doesn't. If we can have a world where women beat themselves up just that little bit less then I feel I've made the impact I wanted to with this part of the book.

Not the End

Over the last few years I have attended seminars with some of the best brains in the business, which has enabled me to accomplish some pretty big things. Rewind only a handful of years and I was the nervous personal trainer struggling to get his courage up to ask for a selfie with whoever had taken the seminar. Now, only a few years later, it's me taking the seminars. Sometimes I see how nervous people get talking to me, and I try my best to break down their nerves with banter, a hug or even putting my arm around them, saying it's okay and that I don't bite. I was that exact person when I was the attendee, so I know it well.

When I attended those events there were literally hundreds of other PTs besides me. I attended some of the events alone and I made friends with them for the day. I remember their names, what they looked like, their branding, the lot. I don't know where those trainers are today; I haven't ever seen any of them on social media, and I sometimes wonder what differentiated me from the others. Why have I reached so many people and they haven't? We learned the exact same things, we were only sitting a foot apart. It's not like I was taught one thing and they were taught another.

It was very important for me to put into action what I learned in those seminars. If I didn't, what was the point? When it comes to video content, I'd say I'm in the top quadrant of people who are recognized for their efforts on social media. Now, do you want to know what my first ever video was on? What topic I picked? Popcorn. Yes, that's right – popcorn.

At the seminar, as part of one of the tasks, I promised myself that the very next day I'd record my first ever video for social media. After spending an hour walking round the flat, looking in cupboards for something – anything – to talk about, I found a bag of popcorn. I was awkward, I stuttered, I wasn't sure what to say. I used my old MacBook's front camera. The quality was awful; the content was worse. I thought I could talk about popcorn being a good low-calorie snack. I waffled on for a few minutes and then saved the video, which nearly killed my laptop and I uploaded it to Facebook to my couple of hundred followers. I think it maybe got about three likes, and they were probably just sympathy likes from family or friends.

I'd go as far to say that video was not only quite embarrassing in hindsight, but also easily **the most important piece of social-media content I have ever created or ever will**.

You see, what I said wasn't important. How I recorded it wasn't important. **It was the sole fact that I had taken action on what I had learned the previous day.** I had gone home and said that tomorrow, without fail, I am recording a video. Could it have been better recorded? Sure. A better topic? Of course. But I took action, and to this day, I am so grateful that I woke up on that Sunday with that attitude. I also had a gut feeling that most of the attendees in the seminars would have woken up the next day and done nothing. If you see my videos now, you could conclude that I am, perhaps, a natural on camera, but I wasn't then. I merely improved by very small fractions behind the scenes for years. My editing, equipment and strategy improved, like an Olympic lifter only ever looking for tiny margins and small incremental improvements each day – not expecting to wake up with extra plates on the bar, just a little better here and there, looking for the long-term return and never getting deflated about the short term.

Ultimately, this book is going to be a waste of time and money for you unless you implement what I have taught you.

The beginning doesn't have to be perfect. Mine certainly wasn't. But over the next few weeks, months, years, you'll need only to search for these small improvements.

Don't be fooled by the next big method that comes your way. You know it's going to be bullshit. Someone's 'secrets to fat loss' or exercise that helps you 'tone up' are all leading to the principle, the calorie deficit. All fat loss that's ever occurred is because of the calorie deficit created, whether the person has known it or not. So ensure that no one around you is being taken advantage of or misled by the zealots and big organizations looking to make a few quid from dressing up the principle as some magical solution.

What gets measured gets improved; logging your food is a powerful short-term tool to bolster your knowledge – if you have any chance of being more intuitive with how much you're eating, this will help. I want you to think of it like tracing paper: we don't need it there for ever, just to improve our habits day by day. One day, eventually, the paper will be removed and your writing will be neater and more balanced. Each person takes a different amount of time developing their writing skills, but there's not a lot that can be done outside repetition and striving for small continual improvements.

Tracking your NEAT is again something to definitely consider should you want to strive to be the most active. Remember, workouts don't burn as many calories as you think, and skipping the odd workout is okay. There are bigger fish to fry, and forcing a workout that you should have skipped helps no one. Try to keep your NEATUP247 whenever possible too.

There are no good or bad **habits**, only ones that play into your ultimate goal and those that don't. Successful people and those who accomplish nothing have the same goals; it's not the goals that are to blame, but the daily habits and processes that mean the most. Where you are going is always much more important than where you currently are.

You need to pay close attention to your life outside of dieting and training. Life is far too fucking short not to have a career you cherish and love. Go after your passion, even if it means moving back in with your parents – because, ultimately, there's a disease out there that's killing the souls of millions, and that's boredom with a payslip attached to it.

The people in your life are very important. Remember the sunk-cost fallacy: the amount of time you've been with someone is not a reason to stay with them even longer. If your partner doesn't support you and your ambitions fully, they're going to cause drag and you don't need that. If you're even considering it, you need to do it. **If it's not a fuck yes, then it's a no.** Human beings instinctively don't like change or being alone – but, ultimately, being selfish and self-centred is an important part of growing, and that's sometimes the identity you need to acquire to do well. You need to be unapologetically yourself, it's empowering. You can't try to please everyone. So say what you're thinking, and don't be afraid or worried about what other people will think.

I hope to have connected many dots that were not connected before for you. I hope to have given you a different perspective, and, at the same time, helped you to look at and audit how you act, who is in your life and why, what you value and what you don't. I hope to have armed you with the knowledge you need so that people can't trick you, fool you or take advantage of you. I need you to pass this forward to people around you too: your friends, colleagues and your family. You should, by now, be better educated than most personal trainers and, unfortunately, a lot of dietitians I have come across. Don't underestimate the power of passing on what you've learned about energy balance, fat loss, female physiology, differentiating diabetes, sleep and much more. You now have the potential power to change the lives around you for the better. If everyone does that after turning the last page in this book, I honestly feel we can change the world and better the lives of the people in it.

I can't do all this for you. I've done my part. From here on in, it's all down to you. You can reread this book and listen to my podcasts to help you stay on track, but it's still down to you. You might go to bed tonight the same, but tomorrow you need to wake up a slightly different person. Someone who is in control of their training, in control of their diet, who gets adequate sleep and balances out their weekends into the week.

You're going to have some awkward conversations, upset some people who get easily offended, and you may even lose a few friends when you rub them up the wrong way with your progress. You may have to tell your employer you're going to leave soon (and you may need a haircut for the interviews you'll be going on).

You have everything you need from this book to go it alone and succeed.

Tomorrow your new identity begins. Be the person who goes after their dreams, rather than just thinking about them, hoping they'll happen. You're armed with the knowledge so that you don't get easily sidetracked or misled on your journey. You'll have realized now that this book wasn't about recipes, home workouts or the bloody benefits of an avocado – it's about self-development and self-help and, if used correctly, it can be a life-altering book.

So just remember: **this is not a diet book**. It's a call-to-action book. It's about empowerment, and you must begin that the second you turn this final page. I'm already excited for you. I'd like to think I'm living proof of the extraordinary things you can achieve in a short period of time when you reset your attitude and ethos, and implement what you've read in these chapters in your daily life.

What you accomplish over the next days, months and even coming years will be a direct result of what you do after closing this book. So, from me, all the best and good luck. The train is about to leave, so make sure you get on it.

James

References

Part I

p.20 Ferriss, Tim, *The 4-Hour Work Week: Escape the 9–5, Live Anywhere and Join the New Rich*, Vermilion (2011)

p.45 *Study: The Effects of Overfeeding on Body Composition: The Role of Macronutrient Composition – A Narrative Review*

p.75, 77 Clear, James, *Atomic Habits: An Easy and Proven Way to Build Good Habits and Break Bad Ones*, Random House (2018)

p.89 Penckofer, S., Byrn, M., Adams, W., Emanuele, M.A., Mumby, P., Kouba, J. and Wallis, D.E., 'Vitamin D supplementation improves mood in women with Type 2 diabetes', *Journal of Diabetes Research*, September 2017: https://www.ncbi.nlm.nih.gov/pmc/articles/PMC5610883/

p.93 Trace, S.E., Thornton, L.M., Runfola, C.D., Lichtenstein, P., Pedersen, N.L. and Bulik, C.M., 'Sleep problems are associated with binge eating in women', *International Journal of Eating Disorders*, July 2012, 45 95), pp.695–703: https://www.ncbi.nlm.nih.gov/pmc/articles/PMC3357460/

p.93 Leproult, R. and Van Cauter, E., 'Effect of 1 week of sleep restriction on testosterone levels in young healthy men', The Journal of the American Medical Association, June 2011, 305 (21): 2173 2174: https://www.ncbi.nlm.nih.gov/pmc/articles/PMC4445839/

p.94 Corona, G., Sforza, A. and Maggi, M., 'Testosterone replacement therapy: long-term safety and efficacy', *The World Journal of Men's Health*, August 2017, 35 (2), pp.65–76: https://www.ncbi.nlm.nih.gov/pubmed/28497912

p.98 Tordjman, S., Chokron, S., Delorme, R., Charrier, A., Bellissant, E., Jaafari, N. and Fougerou, C., 'Melatonin: pharmacology, functions and therapeutic benefits', *Current Neuropharmacology*, April 2017, 15 (3), pp.434–43: https://www.ncbi.nlm.nih.gov/pmc/articles/PMC5405617/

p.99, 105 Walker, Matthew, *Why We Sleep: The New Science of Sleep and Dreams*, Penguin (2018)

p.100 Medic, G., Wille, M. and Hemels, M.E.H, 'Short- and long-term health consequences of sleep disruption', *Nature and Science of Sleep*, May 2017, 9, pp.151–161: https://www.ncbi.nlm.nih.gov/pmc/articles/PMC5449130/

p.102 Southward, K., Rutherfurd-Markwick, K.J. and Ali, A., 'The effect of acute caffeine ingestion on endurance performance: a systematic review and meta-analysis', *Sports Medicine*, August 2018, 48 (8), pp.1913–28: https://www.ncbi.nlm.nih.gov/pubmed/29876876

p.105 Lee, S., Matsumori, K., Nishimura, K., Ikeda, Y., Eto, T. and Higuchi, S., 'Melatonin suppression and sleepiness in children exposed to blue-enriched white LED

lighting at night', *Physiological Reports*, December 2018, 6 (24): https://www.ncbi.
nlm.nih.gov/pmc/articles/PMC6295443/

p.105 For more information on sleep apnoea, see: http://www.sleep-apnoea-trust.org/
driving-and-sleep-apnoea/detailed-guidance-to-uk-drivers-with-sleep-apnoea/

p.106 Nedeltcheva, A.V., Kilkus, J.M., Imperial, J., Schoeller, D.A., Penev, P.D., 'Insufficient
sleep undermines dietary efforts to reduce adiposity', *Annals of Internal Medicine*,
October 2010, 153 (7), pp.435–41: https://www.ncbi.nlm.nih.gov/
pubmed/20921542

p.117 Graham, Phil, *The Diabetic Muscle and Fitness Guide*, Phil Graham (2016). See also
www.diabeticmuscleandfitness.com

p.121 Kahneman, Daniel, *Thinking, Fast and Slow*, Penguin (2012)

p.121 Dobelli, Rolf, *The Art of Thinking Clearly: Better Thinking, Better Decisions*, Sceptre
(2014)

p.129, 144 Manson, Mark, *The Subtle Art of Not Giving a F*ck: A Counterintuitive Approach
to Living a Good Life*, Harper (2016)

p.151 Ferriss, Tim, *Tools of Titans: The Tactics, Routines and Habits of Billionaires, Icons and
World-class Performers*, Vermilion (2016)

p.158, 161 Holiday, Ryan, *Ego Is the Enemy: The Fight to Master Our Greatest Opponent*,
Profile (2017)

Part II

p.181 Harari, Yuval Noah, *Sapiens: A Brief History of Humankind*, Vintage (2015)

— *Homo Deus: A Brief History of Tomorrow*, Vintage (2017)

— *21 Lessons for the 21st Century*, Vintage (2019)

p.184 Trexler, E.T., Smith-Ryan, A.E. and Norton, L.E., 'Metabolic adaptation to weight
loss: implications for the athlete', *Journal of the International Society of Sports
Nutrition*, February 2014, 27; 11 (1): 7: https://www.ncbi.nlm.nih.gov/
pubmed/24571926

p.185 Ostendorf, D.M., Caldwell, A.E., Creasy, S.A., Pan, Z., Lyden, K., Bergouignan, A.,
MacLean, P.S., Wyatt, H.R., Hill, J.O., Melanson, E.L. and Catenacci, V.A., 'Physical
activity energy expenditure and total daily energy expenditure in successful weight
loss maintainers', *Obesity*, March 2019, 27 (3), pp.496–504: https://www.ncbi.nlm.nih.
gov/pubmed/30801984

p.192 Kreher, J.B., 'Diagnosis and prevention of overtraining syndrome: an opinion on
education strategies', *Open Access Journal of Sports Medicine*, 2016, 7, pp.115–22:
https://www.ncbi.nlm.nih.gov/pmc/articles/PMC5019445/

p.194 Thalacker-Mercer, A.E., Fleet, J.C., Craig, B.A., Carnell, N.S. and Campbell, W.W.,
'Inadequate protein intake affects skeletal muscle transcript profiles in older
humans', *The American Journal of Clinical Nutrition*, May 2007, 85 (5), pp.1344–52:
https://www.ncbi.nlm.nih.gov/pubmed/17490972

p.195 Antonio, J., Ellerbroek, A., Silver, T., Vargas, L., Tamayo, A., Buehn, R. and Peacock,
C.A., 'A high-protein diet has no harmful effects: a one-year crossover study in
resistance-trained males', *Journal of Nutrition and Metabolism*, October 2016: https://
www.ncbi.nlm.nih.gov/pubmed/27807480

p.200 Grgic, J., Schoenfeld, B.J. and Latella, C., 'Resistance training frequency and
skeletal muscle hypertrophy: a review of available evidence', *Journal of Science and*

Medicine in Sport, March 2019, 22 (3), pp.361–370: https://www.ncbi.nlm.nih.gov/pubmed/30236847

p.203, 204 Campbell, B.I, Colquhoun, R.J., Zito, G., Martinez, N., Kendall, K., Buchanan, L., Lehn, M., Johnson, M., St Louis, C., Smith, Y. and Cloer, B., 'The effects of a fat loss supplement on resting metabolic rate and hemodynamic variables in resistance trained males: a randomized, double-blind, placebo-controlled, cross-over trial', *Journal of the International Society of Sports Nutrition*, April 2016, 1; 13: 14: https://www.ncbi.nlm.nih.gov/pubmed/27042166

p.204 Rutherfurd-Markwick, K.J. and Ali, A., 'The effect of acute caffeine ingestion on endurance performance: a systematic review and meta-analysis', *Sports Medicine*, August 2018, 48 (8), pp.1913–28: https://www.ncbi.nlm.nih.gov/pubmed/29876876

p.208 Cooper, R., Naclerio, F., Allgrove, J. and Jiminez, A., 'Creatine supplementation with specific view to exercise/sports performance: an update', *Journal of the International Society of Sports Nutrition*, July 2012, 9 (33): https://jissn.biomedcentral.com/articles/10.1186/1550-2783-9-33

p.208 McMorris, T., Harris, R.C., Swain, J., Corbett, J., Collard, K., Dyson, R.J., Dye, L., Hodgson, C. and Draper, N., 'Effect of creatine supplementation and sleep deprivation, with mild exercise, on cognitive and psychomotor performance, mood state, and plasma concentrations of catecholamines and cortisol', *Psychopharmacology*, March 2006, 185 (1), pp.93–103: https://www.ncbi.nlm.nih.gov/pubmed/16416332

p.208 Jagim, A.R., Stecker, R.A., Harty, P.S., Erickson, J.L. and Kerksick, C.M., 'Safety of creatine supplementation in active adolescents and youth: a brief review', *Frontiers In Nutrition*, 2018, 5:15: https://www.ncbi.nlm.nih.gov/pmc/articles/PMC6279854/

p.212 Dieter, B.P., Schoenfeld, B.J. and Aragon, A.A., 'The data do not seem to support a benefit to BCAA supplementation during periods of caloric restriction', *Journal of the International Society of Sports Nutrition*, May 2016, 11 (13). 21: https://www.ncbi.nlm.nih.gov/pubmed/27175106

p.213 Rogerson, D., 'Vegan diets: practical advice for athletes and exercisers', *Journal of the International Society of Sports Nutrition*, December 2017, 14 (1): 36: https://www.researchgate.net/publication/319696943_Vegan_diets_Practical_advice_for_athletes_and_exercisers

p.214 Keithley, J.K., Swanson, B., Mikolaitis, S.L., DeMeo, M., Zeller, J. M., Fogg, L. and Adamji, J., 'Safety and efficacy of glucomannan for weight loss in overweight and moderately obese adults', *Journal of Obesity*, 2013: https://www.ncbi.nlm.nih.gov/pubmed/24490058

p.217 Magnuson, B.A., Carakostas, M.C., Moore, N.H., Poulos, S.P. and Renwick, A.G., 'Biological fate of low-calorie sweeteners', *Nutrition Reviews*, November 2016, 74 (11), pp.670–689: https://www.ncbi.nlm.nih.gov/pubmed/27753624

p.217 Ruiz-Ojeda, F.J., Plaza-Diaz, J., Sáez-Lara, M.J. and Gil, A., 'Effects of sweeteners on the gut microbiota: a review of experimental studies and clinical trials', *Advances in Nutrition*, January 2019, 10 (supplement 1), pp.31–48: https://www.ncbi.nlm.nih.gov/pubmed/30721958

p.218 Müller, M.J., Bosy-Westphal, A. and Heymsfield, S.B., 'Is there evidence for a set point that regulates human body weight?' *F1000 Medicine Reports*, August 2010, 2 (59): https://www.ncbi.nlm.nih.gov/pubmed/21173874

p.221 Anderson, J.W., Konz, E.C., Frederich, R.C. and Wood, C.L., 'Long-term weight-loss maintenance: a meta-analysis of US studies', The American Journal of Clinical Nutrition, November 2001, 74 (5), pp.579–84: https://www.ncbi.nlm.nih.gov/pubmed/11684524

p.227 Schoenfeld, B.J., Aragon, A.A., Wilborn, C.D., Krieger, J.W. and Sonmez, G.T., 'Body composition changes associated with fasted versus non-fasted aerobic exercise', Journal of International Society of Sports Nutrition, November 2014, 18; 11 (1): 54: https://www.ncbi.nlm.nih.gov/pubmed/25429252

p.229 Park, S., Ahn, J. and Lee, B., 'Very-low-fat diets may be associated with increased risk of metabolic syndrome in the adult population', Clinical Nutrition, October 2016, 35 (5), pp.1159–1167: https://www.sciencedirect.com/science/article/abs/pii/S0261561415002447

p.230 Tipton, K.D., Hamilton, D.L. and Gallagher, I.J., 'Assessing the role of muscle protein breakdown in response to nutrition and exercise in humans', Sports Medicine, March 2018, 48 (supplement 1), pp.53–64: https://www.ncbi.nlm.nih.gov/pubmed/29368185

p.231, 236 Hall, K.D. and Guo, J., 'Obesity energetics: body weight regulation and the effects of diet composition', Gastroenterology, May 2017, 152 (7), pp.1718–1727: https://www.ncbi.nlm.nih.gov/pubmed/28193517

p.241 Sievert, K., Hussain, S.M., Page, M.J., Wang, Y., Hughes, H.J., Malek, M. and Cicuttini, F.M., 'Effect of skipping breakfast on subsequent energy intake: systematic review and meta-analysis of randomized controlled trials', The BMJ, January 2019, 364:142: https://www.ncbi.nlm.nih.gov/pubmed/30700403

p.245 Allen, M., Dickinson, K.M. and Prichard, I., 'The dirt on clean eating: a cross sectional analysis of dietary intake, restrained eating and opinions about clean eating among women', Nutrients, Spetember 2018, 10 (9), p.ii: https://www.ncbi.nlm.nih.gov/pubmed/30205540

p.251 Bagherniya, M., Butler, A.E., Barreto, G.E. and Sahebkar, A., 'The effect of fasting or calorie restriction on autophagy induction: A review of the literature', Ageing Research Reviews, November 2018, 47: https://www.ncbi.nlm.nih.gov/pubmed/30172870

p.273 Unfer, V., Facchinetti, F., Orrù, B., Giordani, B. and Nestler, J., 'Myo-inositol effects in women with PCOS: a meta-analysis of randomized controlled trials', Endocrine Connections, November 2017, 6 (8), pp.647–658: https://www.ncbi.nlm.nih.gov/pubmed/29042448

p.276, 277 Kominiarek, M. A. and Rajan, P., 'Nutrition recommendations in pregnancy and lactation', Medical Clinics of North America, November 2016, 100 (6), pp.1199–1215: https://www.ncbi.nlm.nih.gov/pmc/articles/PMC5104202/

Acknowledgements

I need to give a special thank you firstly to my clients, all of them, and especially the JSA members who have put their trust in me over the years and allowed me to live a life where I've had the time and capacity to read so much more, and even write my own book. Without their trust and faith in me there would not be a book in front of you today.

Thank you to HarperCollins UK for being audacious, brave and willing enough to sign me as a first-time author. Special thank you to Lydia, Oli and Orlando for putting a vision into a hardback book.

Words could not describe my continued gratitude to my family, who over the years have supported me through thick and thin. I don't tell them enough so here it is in writing, in a book, of all things. Life isn't always easy and the support from my family has been second to none, from my sister lending me her lunch money when I was at school all the way to seeking refuge from my very busy work schedule at my parents' house – and all they ask in return is that I throw a tennis ball for the dog and cook on the barbecue.

A big thank you to Ben Carpenter and Martin MacDonald for being my go-to resources in times of need. And a special mention to Ben for contributing and directing me in many parts of the book to relevant sources, with an impeccable response time on WhatsApp.

My friends have been the pillars of my mental health since my first day of becoming a personal trainer, so a huge thank you to Diren, Jayde, Holden and Perry. All of this would have felt a lot like work without your continued support.

Lucy Lord, #notmybird, thank you. We baked a cake when I had 10,000 followers and we sat back thinking I'd completed life. Your positivity and support has been a huge contributor to everything I currently have.

Last but certainly not least, thank you, Luke. A man with a vision for what I could accomplish and the belief to back me from the very early days. A manager, my events guy, but now also one of my best friends. The man in the shadows who took my dreams and aspirations and made them my reality.

Thank you!

Without you lot, I very much doubt we'd be here with a book.

A special thank you to the following peers, friends and experts who have helped to inform the research-based analysis within this book:

- Ben Carpenter @bdccarpenter
- Bret Contreras @bretcontreras1
- Martin MacDonald @martinnutrition
- Menno Henselmans @menno.henselmans
- Phil Graham @philgraham01
- Sohee Lee @soheefit

Further Reading

Here are just a few of my top reading recommendations for inspiration and empowerment:

Bergeron, Ben, *Chasing Excellence: A Story About Building the World's Fittest Athletes*, Lioncrest Publishing (2017)

Clear, James, *Atomic Habits: An Easy and Proven Way to Build Good Habits and Break Bad Ones*, Random House (2018)

Ferriss, Timothy, *The 4-Hour Work Week: Escape the 9–5, Live Anywhere and Join the New Rich*, Vermillion (2011)

Harari, Yuval Noah, *Sapiens: A Brief History of Humankind*, Vintage (2015)

Holiday, Ryan, *Ego is the Enemy: The Fight to Master Our Greatest Opponent*, Profile Books (2017)

Holiday, Ryan, *Stillness is the Key: An Ancient Strategy for Modern Life*, Profile Books (2019)

Holiday, Ryan, *The Obstacle is the Way: The Ancient Art of Turning Adversity into Opportunity*, Profile Books (2015)

Index

amenorrhoea (discontinuation of
menstrual cycle) 268–70
artificial sweeteners 215–17
autophagy 238, 250–2

BCAAs (Branched Chain Amino
Acids) 210–12, 213
BMR (basal metabolic rate) 59,
60–1, 70, 163, 183, 184, 272
body fat, measuring 54–8
Brazilian jiu jitsu (BJJ) 66, 77, 97,
100, 140, 156–7, 178
breakfast 28, 29, 66, 211, 238–41,
242, 248–9, 250, 251
breastfeeding 276–8
'bro split' (separating training into
certain body parts allocating
an entire day to them)
197–202

calorie deficit, the 37–58
body fat, measuring and 54–8
calorie calculators 47–9
disputing/confirmation bias 42–6
'hunger hormones' (leptin and
ghrelin) 40–1
weight and 52–4
calories in calories out (CICO) 42,
43

carbohydrates 27–8
cheat meals 221–5
clean eating 241–5
coffee 53, 100, 101, 109, 214, 239,
249, 250
comparison and choice, progress
and 14–18
confirmation bias 44–6, 120–1, 175
consumer-method-principle
25–6, 33
creatine 65, 206, 207–9
CrossFit 61, 126, 188, 236, 255

diabetes 111–17
defined 112–16
insulin resistance and 115
treatment of 117
type I 113–14
type II 114

ectomorph 171, 172, 172, 177
effort 139–45, 149–57
endomorph 171, 172, 172, 176, 177
exercise activity thermogenesis
(EAT) 61–2, 63, 69, 184
exercising, training vs 253–60

fasted cardio 14, 121, 226–7, 249
fat burners 203–5

fat loss:
  female 261–78
  muscle gain and 33–6
  sleep and 106–9
fitness events 11–14
fitness fallacies 181–260
fitness industry:
  fitness events and 11–14
  future of 8–9
  right now 4–7
fitness tracking 67–9, 70, 185
5:2 diet 26, 273
flexible dieting 82–5

goal setting 152–7

habits 73–85
  flexible dieting 82–5
  IIFYM ('If it fits your macros
    movement') 78–81
  'hunger hormones' (leptin and
    ghrelin) 40–1

IIFYM ('If it fits your macros') 78–81
impostor syndrome 164–7
insulin resistance 114, 115, 116, 229,
    265, 270, 271, 272, 273, 276
intermittent fasting (IF) 28–9,
    246–52
  alertness and fasted state 250
  autophagy and 250–2
  belief system 246–9
  length of 249

ketogenic diet 27–8, 43, 44, 115–16,
    195, 232–3, 234, 235, 237
ketosis 28, 113, 195, 232, 234, 235

leucine 212–13
low-carb diet 18, 27, 28, 39, 43,
    44–5, 46, 121, 228–37, 250
low-fat diet 30, 83, 229, 237

macronutrients 27, 28, 30, 45, 55,
    78–9, 80, 81–2, 83, 172, 184,
    228, 229, 230, 233, 236, 237
menopause 274–6
menstrual cycle 13, 53, 262–8, 269,
    275–6
mesomorph 171, 172, 175, 177
metabolism:
  'body types' and 174–8
  breakfast and 240–1

NEAT (non-exercise activity
    thermogenesis) 63–9
  habits to have 64–7
  #NEATUP247 60, 69, 185, 281
  tracking with fitness trackers
    67–8
non-essential supplementation
    209
non-fat-related fluctuations
    53–4
numbers, power of 131–4

overtraining 188–96

PCOS 49, 115, 263, 268, 269–73
personal-trainer (PT):
  dietitians and 10
  qualifications 8–9, 10, 13, 17, 111
plateau 158–64
polarization 135–8
pregnancy calories 276–8

progressive overload 70, 166, 254,
    257–60, 265
protein:
  BCAAs and 210–13
  benefit of reducing protein to
      create a calorie deficit 230
  daily target 194
  absorption of 195–6
  gluconeogenesis 195
  'muscle protein synthesis' 195,
      212–13, 230, 239
  whey protein 27, 80, 206–7, 209,
      211

16:8/Intermittent fasting (IF)
    28–9
sleep 90–109
  apps 109
  audiobooks/podcasts and 108
  caffeine and 101–2, 108–9
  disruption 100–105
    alcohol 102
    caffeine 101
    drug abuse 102
    jet lag 104
    light 104–5
    shift work 102
  fat loss and 106–9
  hormones, sleep rhythm and
      95–100

magnesium and lavender spray
    109
  overeating and 92–3
  sleep apnoea 105–6
  testosterone and 93–4
slimming clubs 30
somatotypes 171–80
sport selection 178–80
starvation mode 182–7, 203
sunk cost fallacy 121–7, 282
supplements 206–13 see also
    individual supplement name

testosterone replacement therapy
    (TRT) 93–4
thermic effect of food (TEF) 62,
    163, 183, 222, 227
tool belt, lifestyle/goal 70–1, 87,
    176
training vs exercising 253–60

vitamin D 87–9

water weight 46, 53
weight, fat and 52–4
weight-loss shots 214
weight regain 218–21
weight-tracking organizations 30
whey protein 27, 80, 206–7, 209,
    211

If you enjoyed the book and would like to see more of what I can do to help you in the next stage of your journey, feel free to head to the James Smith Academy:

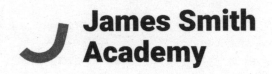

James Smith Academy

www.jamessmithacademy.com
@Jamessmithpt